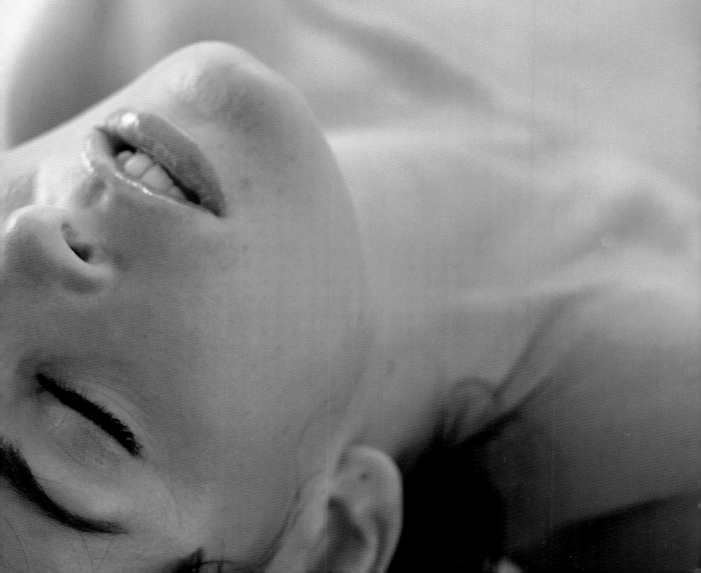

THE
KAMA SUTRA
YEAR

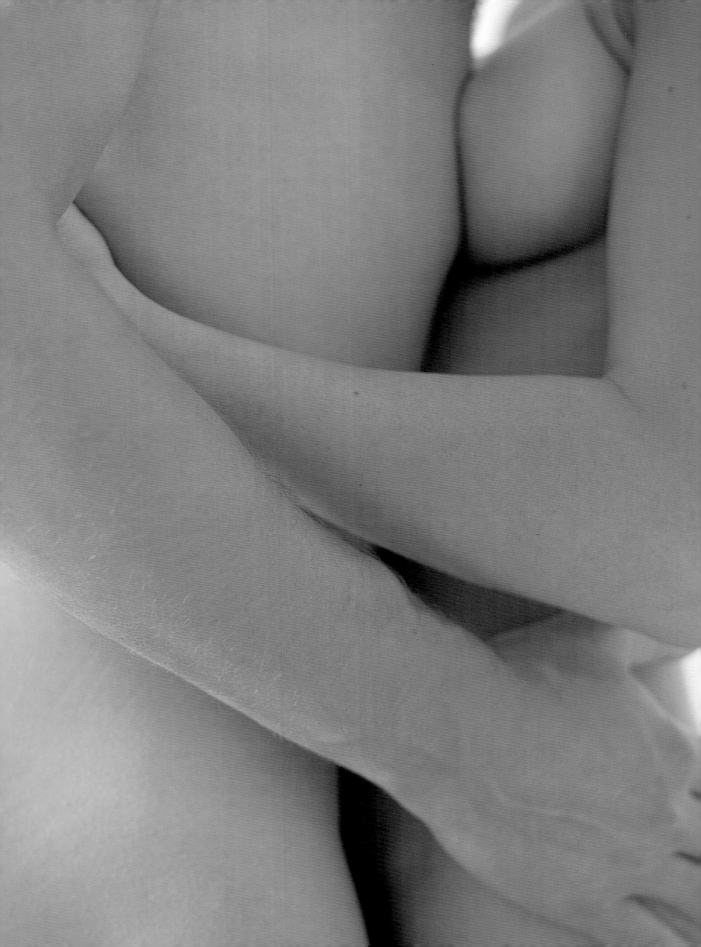

THE KAMA SUTRA YEAR

52 Sensational Positions for Erotic Pleasure

Eleanor McKenzie

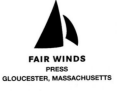

FAIR WINDS
PRESS
GLOUCESTER, MASSACHUSETTS

Text © 2005 Octopus Publishing Group Ltd

First published in the USA in 2005 by
Fair Winds Press
33 Commercial Street
Gloucester, MA 01930

The right of Eleanor McKenzie to be identified as the author of this work has been asserted by her in accordance with the Copyright, Design, and Patents Act, 1988.

08 07 06 05 04   1 2 3 4 5

ISBN 1-59233-105-X

Library of Congress Cataloging-in-Publication Data available

Cover design by Tokiko Morishima
Book design by Joanna MacGregor

Printed and bound in Hong Kong

WARNING
With the prevalence of AIDS and other sexually transmitted diseases, if you do not practice safe sex you are risking your life and your partner's life.

Contents

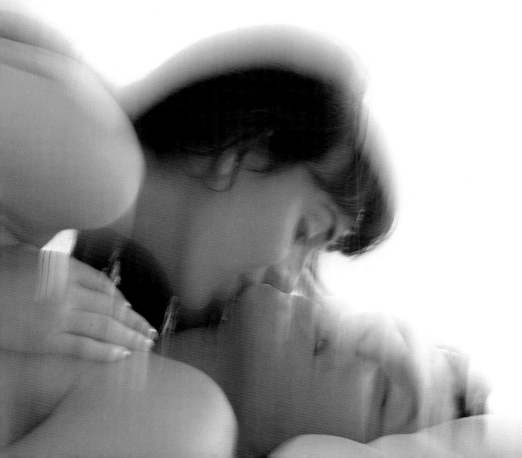

Introduction

Imagine being served the same food every day, or knowing that every Friday night you are going to have the same meal. Before long you will be bored; so bored you won't even want to eat no matter how hungry you are. What then tends to happen is that you start looking for places where you can have the variety that you crave to satisfy your hunger. Sex is food for the mind, body and soul, and we underestimate its importance if we serve up exactly the same dish week in, week out.

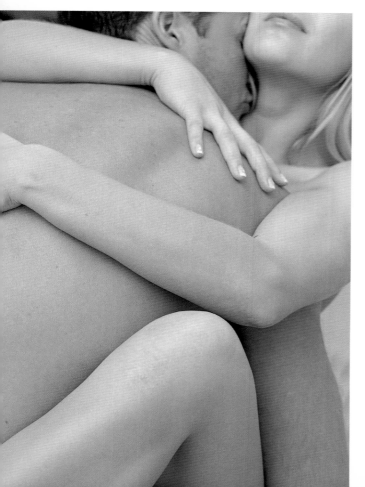

Sexual variety is the essence of a healthy sexual relationship. Nowhere is this more clearly understood than in the ancient love texts of the East, of which the *Kama Sutra* is the most famous.

Kama Sutra means 'science of love'. It is one of the oldest, and certainly the most famous, of texts devoted to the principles of sensual pleasure and was compiled some 2,000 years ago by Mallinaga Vatsyayana, an Indian sage who was living in the holy city of Benares (Varanasi).

Kama (pleasure or sensual gratification) is just one of the three spiritual practices considered necessary for the release of the soul from reincarnation, the other two being *dharma* (virtue or religious merit) and *artha* (worldly wealth). Through the practice of *kama* we are to enjoy the world through our senses as well as our mind and spirit. Sexual pleasure is the chief means of practising *kama*.

The *Kama Sutra* is more than a sex manual; it is a social document about the way courtship, marriage and relationships were conducted in Hindu society.

Because of this, and because of its antiquity, it does not need to be followed precisely by present-day lovers. By all means you can read it for its historical importance, to get the flavour of the period and to be inspired, but its continued importance is as a source for modern interpretation. Think of it as an ancient recipe book with dishes for which some ingredients are no longer available, and we must improvise our recreation of the dishes with what is accessible now. This does not mean we lack the important elements, rather that we have some slightly different additions available, such as a variety of sex toys, videos and the internet to spice things up.

Anywhere can be the kitchen of your sexual creativity, so do not confine yourself to the bedroom; you have other spaces in your home, and there are many more in the world outside. There are no limits on where sex can begin or where you can end up making love. The only limits are imposed by your imagination.

With that in mind, this book offers an assortment of sexual positions derived from the *Kama Sutra*. There are 52 in total – one for every week of the year. Even if you aim to try just one new posture every week, your sexual repertoire will increase, which is the most important point. A little variety, added slowly, is perhaps better than attempting to try everything in one week. Go too fast and you will not give yourself time to explore the sensations of each posture or to master it.

Take your time; discover what works for you. While each posture is fully illustrated and accompanied by a clear step-by-step guide that will enable you to enjoy them all effortlessly, please follow the spirit of the instructions rather than the letter. This book is intended to support and encourage your explorations, not to dictate your journey.

Sex has a variety of moods; thus the positions range from the intimate to the passionate, from the energetic to the tranquil. Whether it is a night of slow, lingering sex or a passionate one that demands something more energetic, lovers will find there is something to suit all their moods and desires.

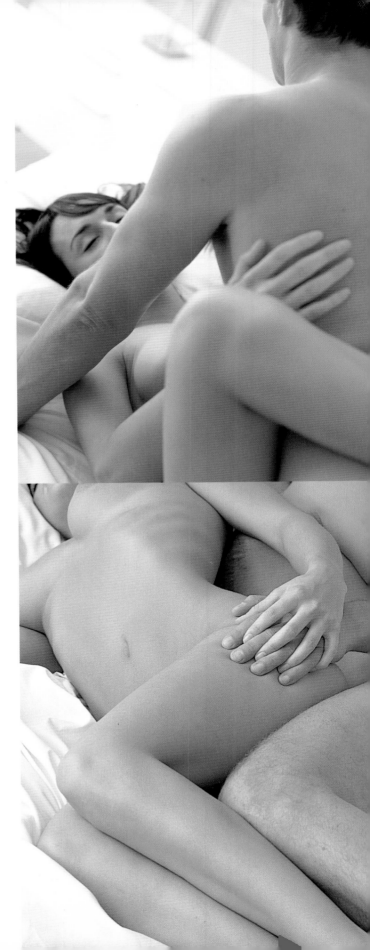

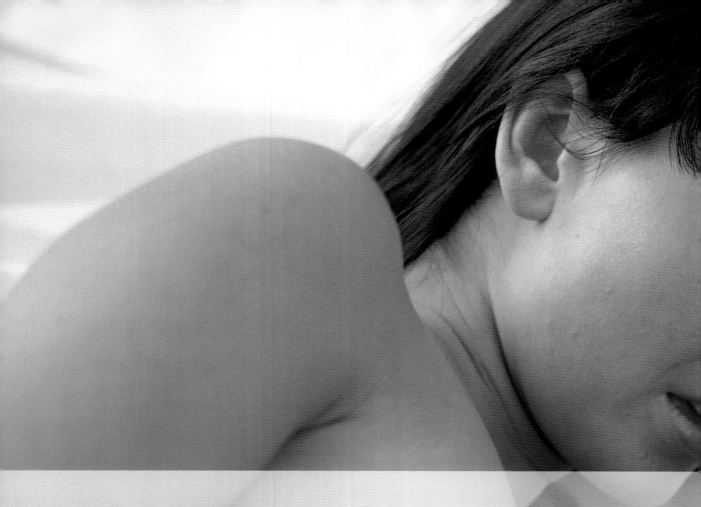

Intimate

Intimacy itself is still and subtle rather than loud and dramatic. Allow yourself to be completely open with your partner, permit them to break through all your defences, and you will enter the blissful union of knowing yourselves as 'one' – the ultimate intimacy about which many teachers have written.

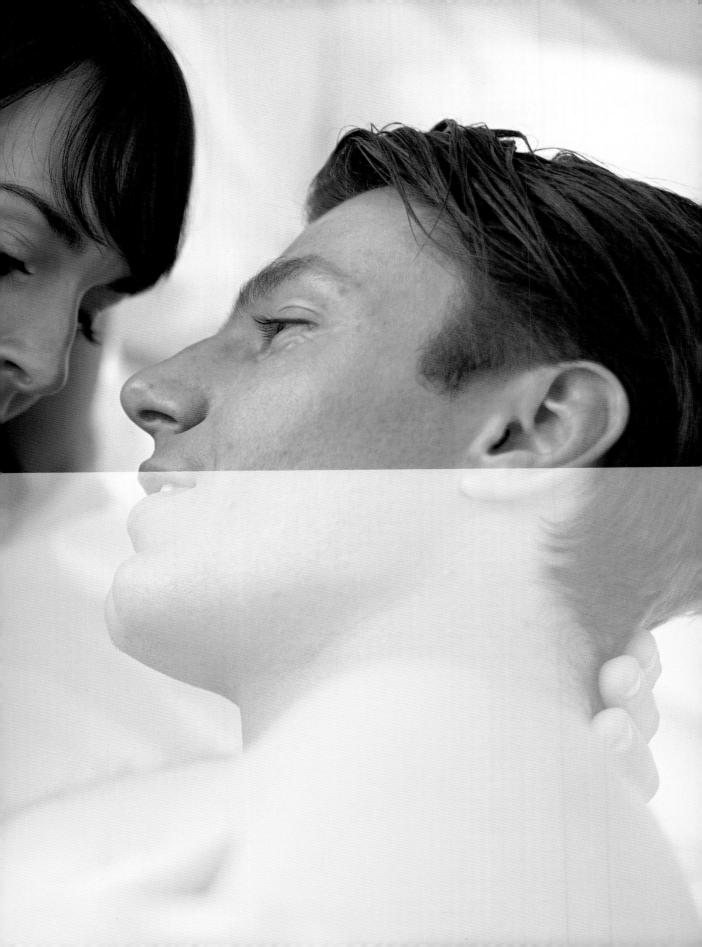

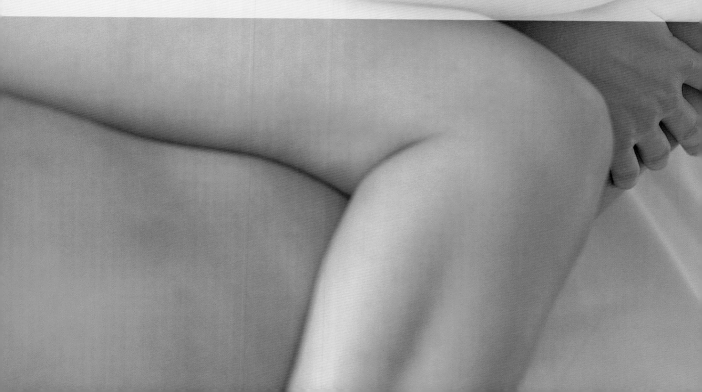

Sesame and rice

An embrace holds us together. In its stillness we may find the first stirrings of desire or a rekindling of it. We may also bathe in its warmth when we have satiated ourselves of our passion. The beauty of an embrace is that it is a shared moment of reflection from which we emerge to face the world both together and separately.

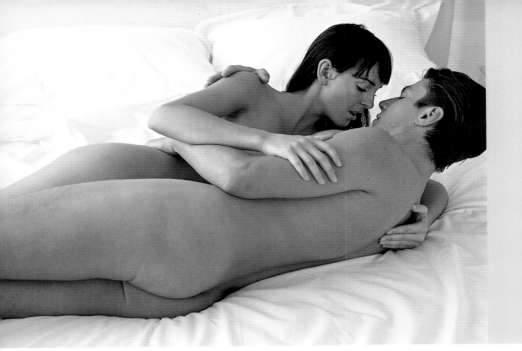

Gain intimacy through a loving embrace whatever time of the day or night. While lying down, turn to face one another and cross your arms loosely around each other's backs.

The woman gently slips her lower leg between the man's thighs and reaches with her other leg over the top of his uppermost thigh, letting it rest there. Their bodies, and their genitals, are now held in a tight embrace.

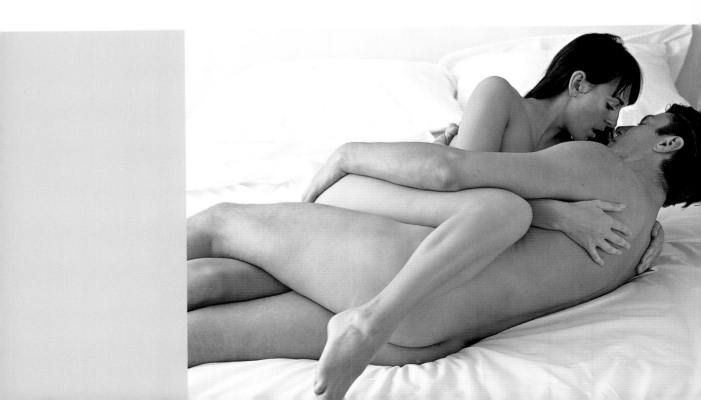

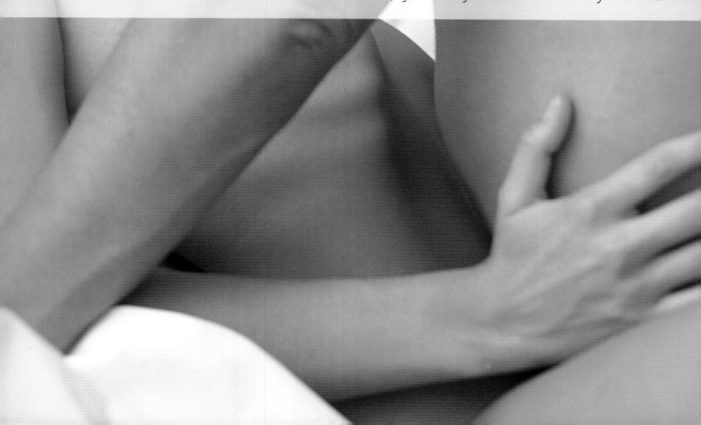

The missionary

Universally known and loved, this face-to-face position provides the all-important intimacy of eye contact. While lying on her back, the woman opens herself to her lover while being protected by his body arching over her; he is the sky that holds itself up as a canopy over the earth, yet they meet on every horizon.

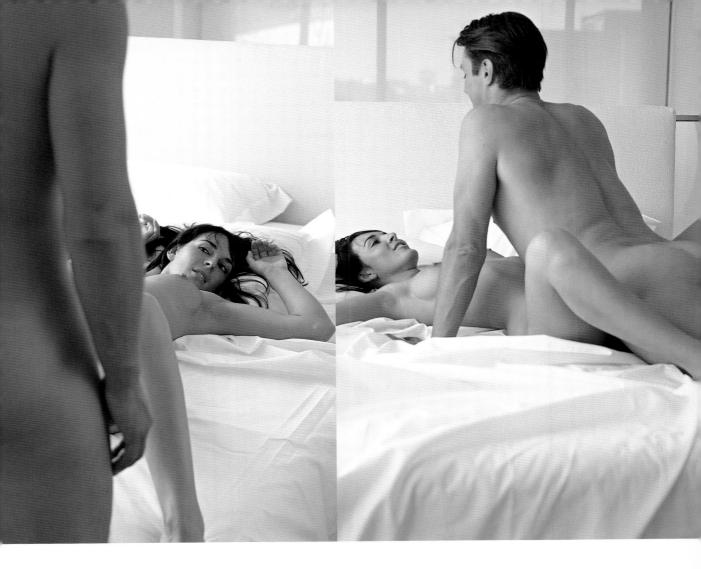

Using plenty of pillows or cushions, if desired, the woman lies on her back and opens her legs, keeping her knees raised and loosely bent and allowing enough space for her lover to lie between them.

The man positions himself between her legs and, holding his penis with one hand, guides it in to her. Once inside her, he supports himself with his fully extended arms so that his weight does not press too heavily on her. Maintaining eye contact throughout heightens the intimacy of this position and both can enjoy the sight of him thrusting into her.

This extremely popular position allows partners to watch each other's pleasure.

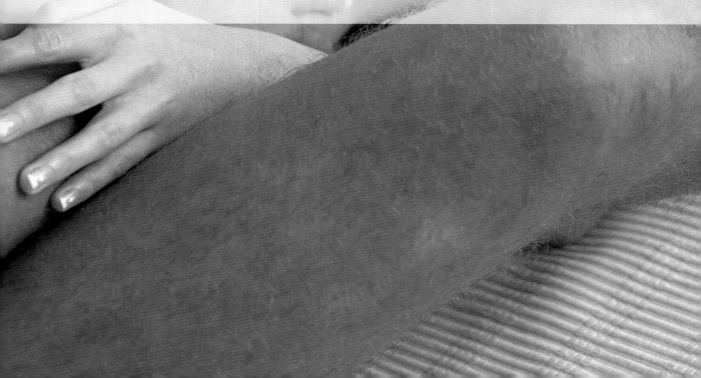

A rose in bloom

This posture offers both deep penetration and relaxation for both lovers. The use of furniture and cushions for support can make it even more restful, especially for the man. This intimate and sensual position also offers an excellent opportunity for the man to manually bring the woman to orgasm during penetration.

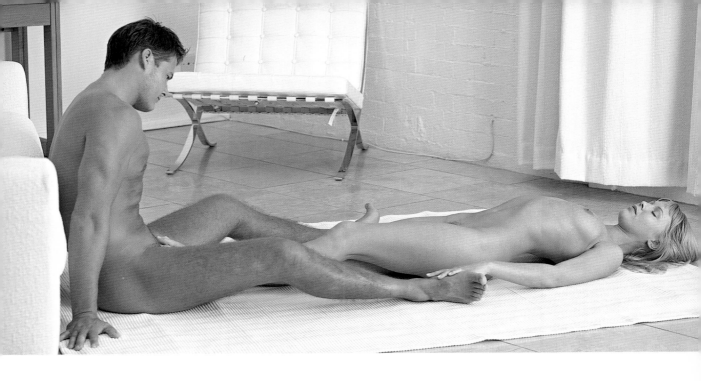

The man sits on the floor with a straight back, opens his legs and lets his knees fall gently outwards, keeping them relaxed. He may well be more comfortable if his back is supported by a sofa, a comfortable chair or the edge of a low bed. The woman lies on her back facing him and takes up the space between his already open legs.

He then gently raises her legs on to his shoulders and penetrates her, pulling her hips towards him and holding her as close to him as possible. They can choose now to stay still briefly, and then find their own rhythm as he holds her hips and moves them in time with his own. This position allows him to play easily with her clitoris and bring her to orgasm that way, if preferred.

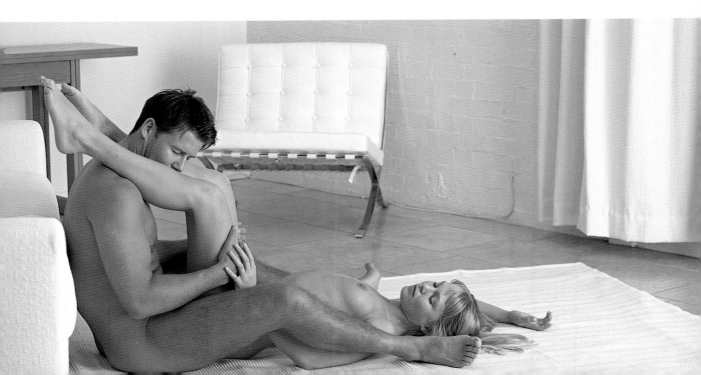

Unicorn's horn

Like the mythical unicorn after which it is named, this slightly athletic position can be magical for both lovers as it provides the stimulation of a snug fit for the penis and, for the man, the visual stimulus of watching his lover's buttocks as she moves on his erection. This position also allows the woman to touch her clitoris during penetration to add to her pleasure.

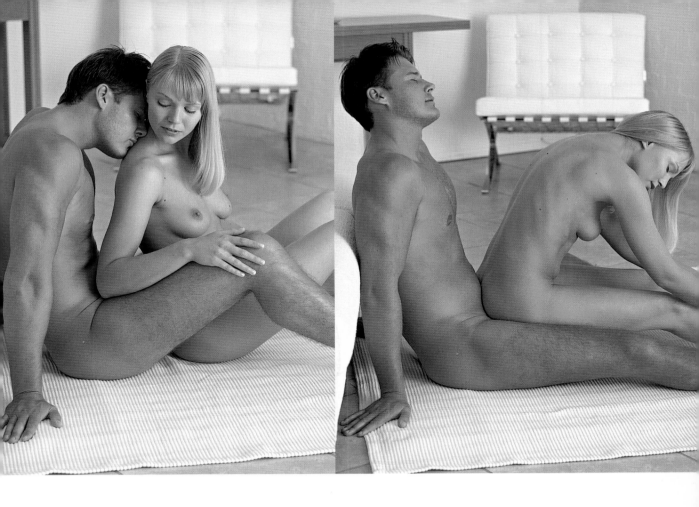

The man sits on the floor with a straight back, ideally supported behind by furniture. He opens his legs, allowing his lover sufficient space to sit between them. With her back to him, the woman lowers herself gently on to him with her legs straight out in front of her. She transfers her weight on to her hands, which are on the floor either side of her legs, so that she can raise her buttocks while he slips his penis inside her. He supports his own weight on his hands.

Now, either lover can provide the movement necessary for stimulation: the man can thrust upwards slightly or he can stay still, and the woman can move her hips in a circular or up-and-down motion. Any movement should be subtle rather than dramatic but, because of the tightness of the vagina in this position, any shift in position will be extremely pleasurable to both partners.

This position can be made even more exciting if it is performed in front of a large floor-length mirror.

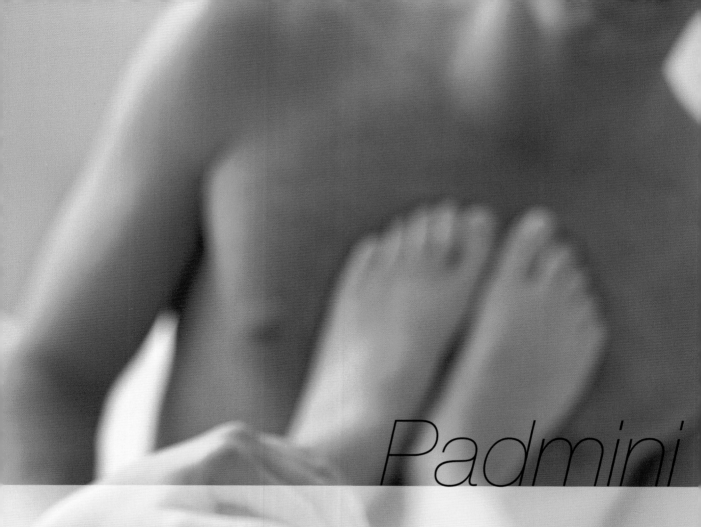

Padmini

In this posture the woman lies on her back with her knees raised – a position where her vagina is both tightened and shortened. Some couples may prefer to use this position for shallow thrusting, to add an element of teasing, with the man allowing only the head of the penis to penetrate the woman.

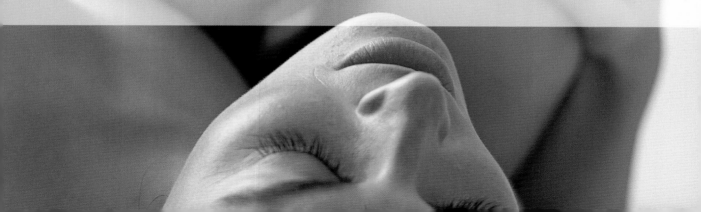

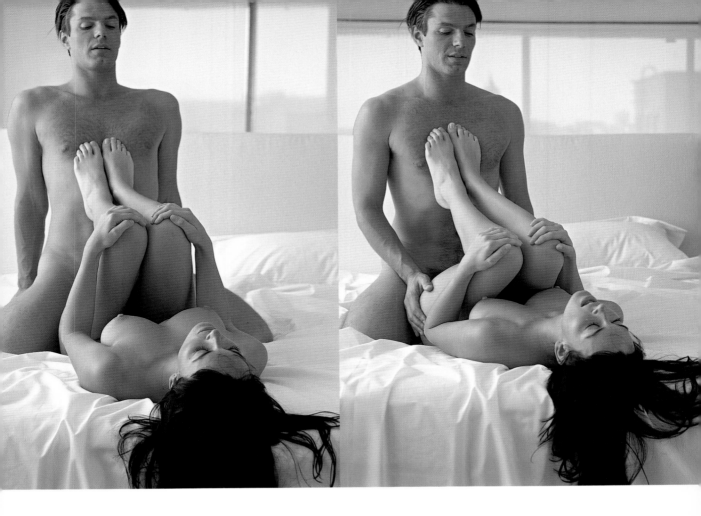

Some couples may find it more pleasurable to use a lubricant of some kind before adopting this posture, to counter the tightness of the vagina. The woman lies on her back and pulls her knees up towards her chest. She then holds them together, using a hand on each knee or, if preferred, crossing her hands over her knees, while keeping her shoulders relaxed. The man kneels in front of her, with his knees on either side of her hips, and penetrates her.

To support herself, the woman moves her feet to rest against his solar plexus. Now, he grasps her hips firmly while moving inside her. This position is ideal to employ the artful style of thrusting – as described in the *Kama Sutra* – that guarantees exquisite pleasure for the woman. In the 'Set of Nine' system, the man does nine shallow thrusts and one deep, then eight shallow thrusts and two deep, and so on, finishing with one shallow thrust and nine deep.

The man controls the movement and depth of thrust, plus he can see his penis moving in and out of her, adding to his excitement.

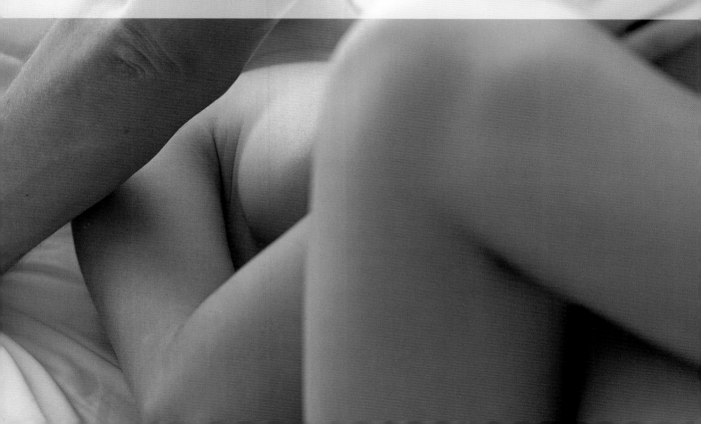

Water crane

Some positions are known to have not only a stimulating but also a healing effect on a woman's internal organs, and this is one of them. The depth of thrusting stimulates the organs in a similar way to acupressure or acupuncture. Thus, the position of the woman's body determines which 'meridian points' the penis stimulates.

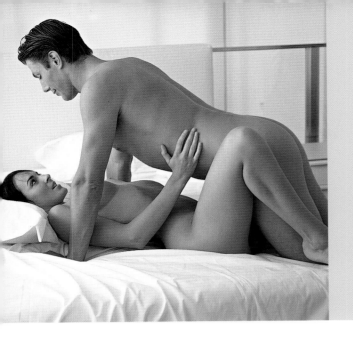

The woman's movement keeps the man erect, while his penis massages her from within.

The woman lies on her back with her head and upper back supported by pillows. When she is comfortable and ready, the man kneels between her legs and folds his body at the hips so that his upper body is parallel with hers. He uses his hands, placed either side of her body, for support.

He then penetrates her, but only shallowly. She lifts her legs and wraps them firmly around his waist to support herself. He then remains still while she rotates her pelvis, first clockwise then anticlockwise, for as long as possible and until orgasms ripple through both their bodies.

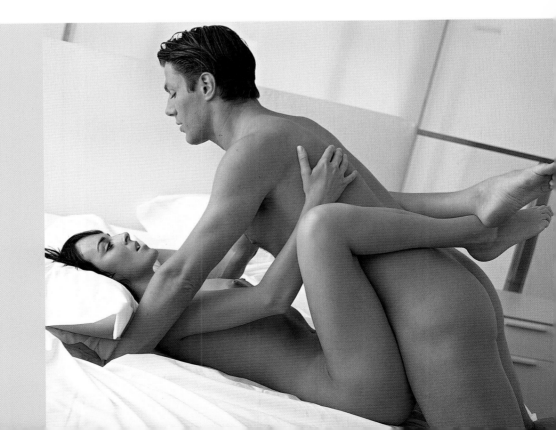

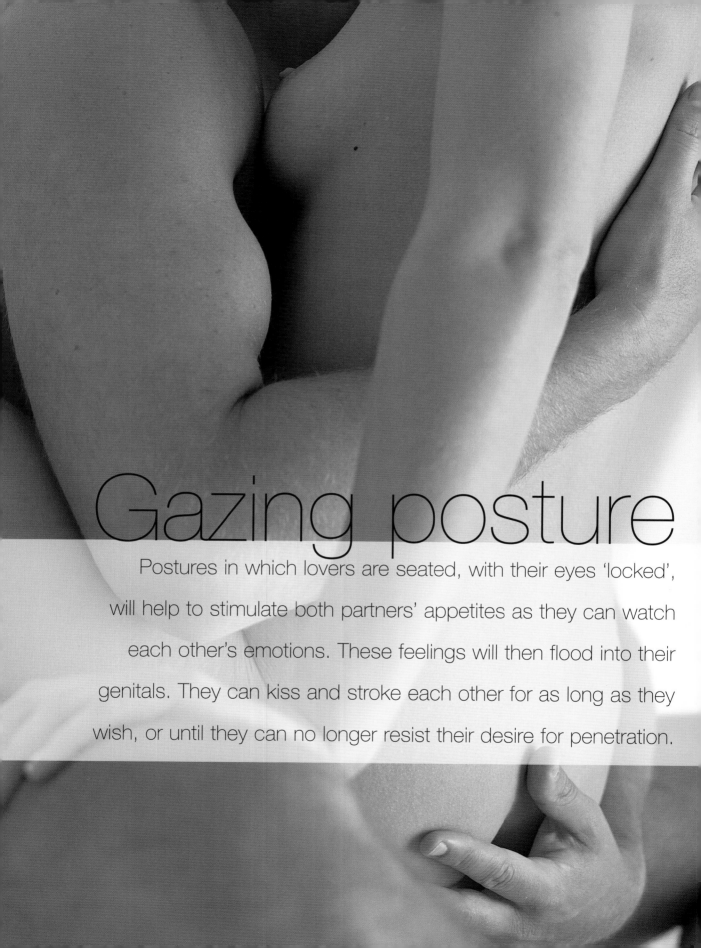

Gazing posture

Postures in which lovers are seated, with their eyes 'locked',
will help to stimulate both partners' appetites as they can watch
each other's emotions. These feelings will then flood into their
genitals. They can kiss and stroke each other for as long as they
wish, or until they can no longer resist their desire for penetration.

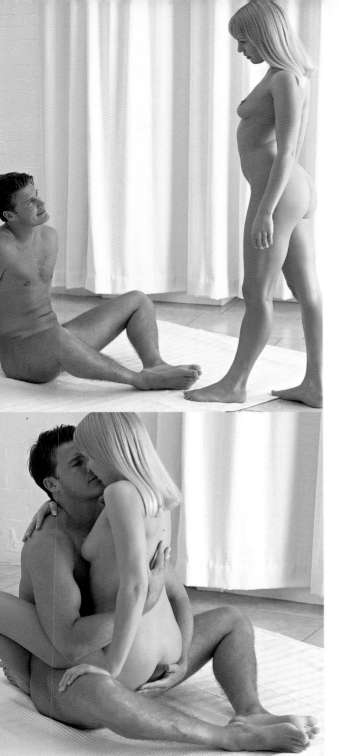

The man sits upright on a rug or large cushion so that he is comfortable. He could also lean against a chair or bed to support his back, if wished. He parts his legs and bends them at the knees, with the soles of his feet touching. In this way he creates a 'seat' for the woman.

The woman straddles him and crosses her legs behind his back, with her arms gently resting behind his shoulders or on his thighs. He supports her lower back and buttocks with his hands. As well as kissing and stroking in this position, the lovers can also gently rub against each other's genitals, arousing each other before attempting penetration. Quietly they can listen to their senses and use this position meditatively for as long as they wish. Alternatively, the man can penetrate the woman immediately but, once he is inside, only the woman should move, making circular or sideways motions with her hips; the man can help her, or at least join in, by directing her hips with his hands.

This close and intimate position can be used with or without penetration, depending on your mood at the time.

Yin yang

This is one of the best positions for 'taking a break' during energetic sex. It is wonderful to get into this position following orgasm, while the man is still relatively hard; then, the woman can either keep him inside for longer or massage the penis into another erection using her vaginal muscles. Once they have rested, the couple can quickly adopt a position where the man can thrust more easily.

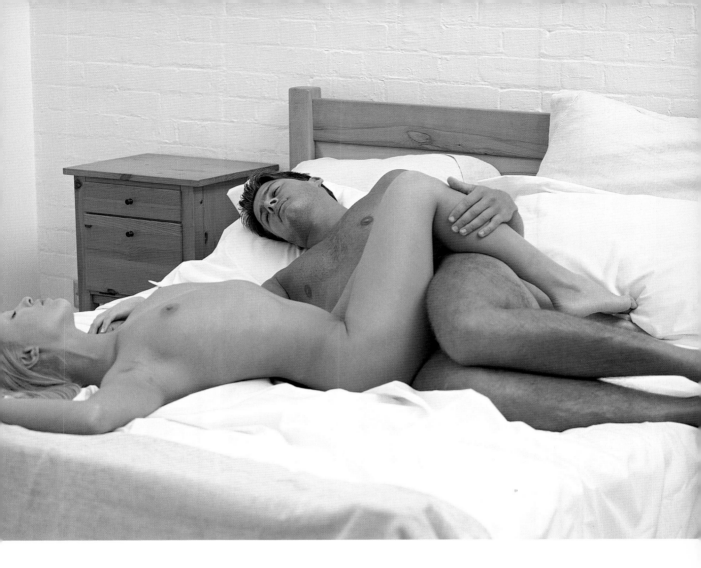

While lying on his side across the bed, the man rests his head on his hand; alternatively he may find it more comfortable to rest his head on a pillow and stretch out his arm instead. The woman gently reclines herself so that she is on her back at right angles to him, with her legs draped over his hips. He rests one arm across her legs while the other holds her hand or fondles another part of her body. In this position, he can penetrate her. Alternatively, they can take up this position while he is already inside her. In either case, this is a position for staying still and the muscles of the woman's vagina are the only ones to move.

This is a beautiful and very intimate position in which to fall asleep after making love.

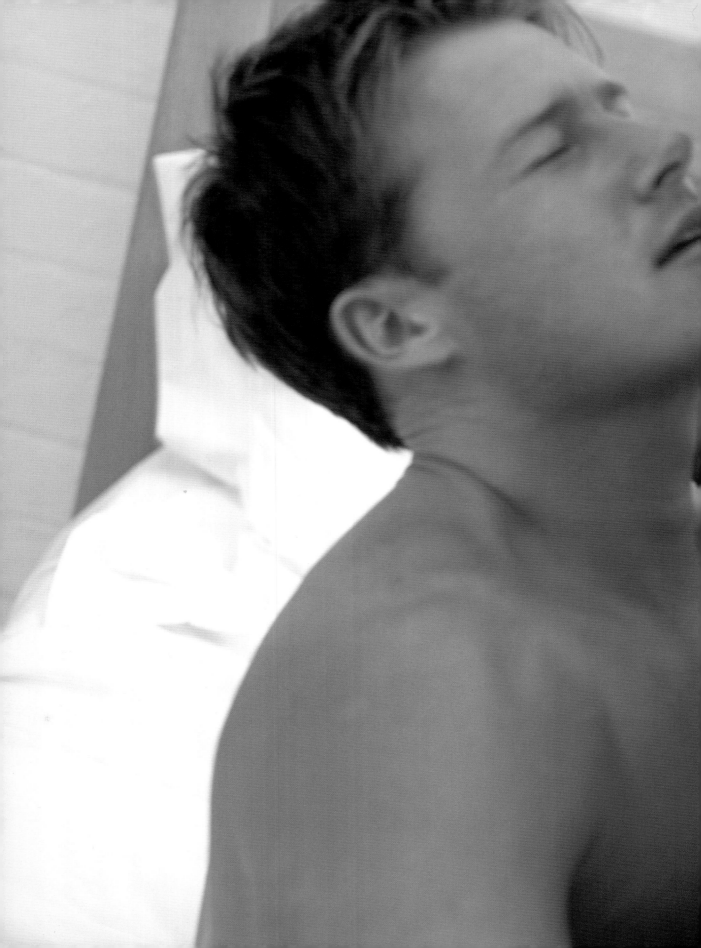

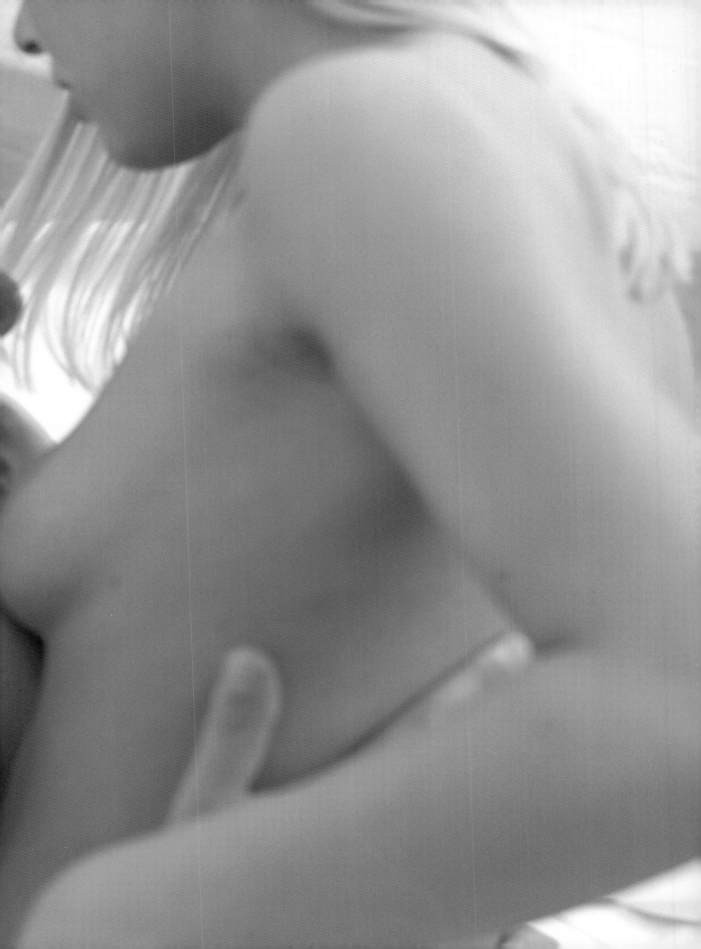

Rolling posture

This face-to-face posture allows penetration, or not, depending on how the lovers feel at the time. One idea would be to start off in the Gazing Posture (see page 22) and, after penetration, to transfer into this Rolling Posture, which allows the woman to alter the tightness and length of her vagina simply by moving her legs slightly. The man plays a part, too, using his hips to create movement and sensation.

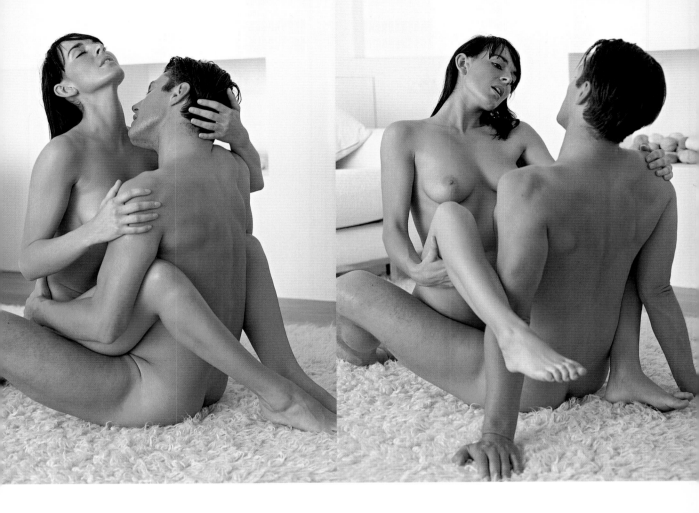

The man sits upright on a rug, large cushion or quilt. He parts his legs and bends them at the knees, with the soles of his feet touching. In this way he creates a 'seat' for the woman. The woman sits facing him, her buttocks cradled by his thighs and her legs wrapped around his back, with her feet resting on the floor.

She bends one leg upwards at his side and holds her hand under her thigh so that she can lift her leg slightly up and down; it is with this subtle shift that she alters the sensations they both experience. She holds on to the man by reaching her other arm around the back of his neck. It is difficult for the woman to make any other movement in this position; however, the man, supported on his hands, can roll his hips from side to side, hence the name of the posture.

Here, slight leg movements control arousal.

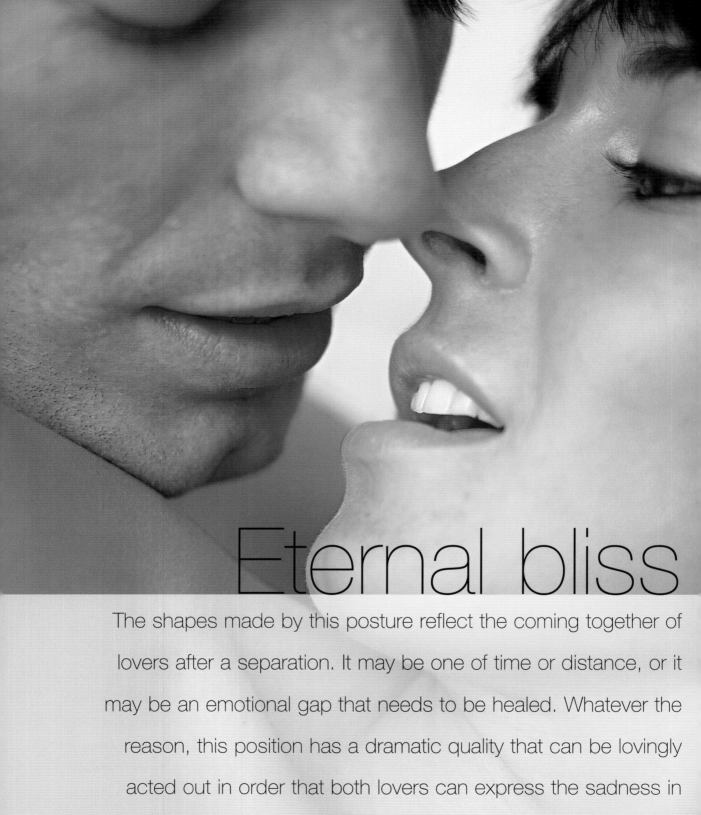

Eternal bliss

The shapes made by this posture reflect the coming together of lovers after a separation. It may be one of time or distance, or it may be an emotional gap that needs to be healed. Whatever the reason, this position has a dramatic quality that can be lovingly acted out in order that both lovers can express the sadness in having been apart and their deeply felt passion at being reunited.

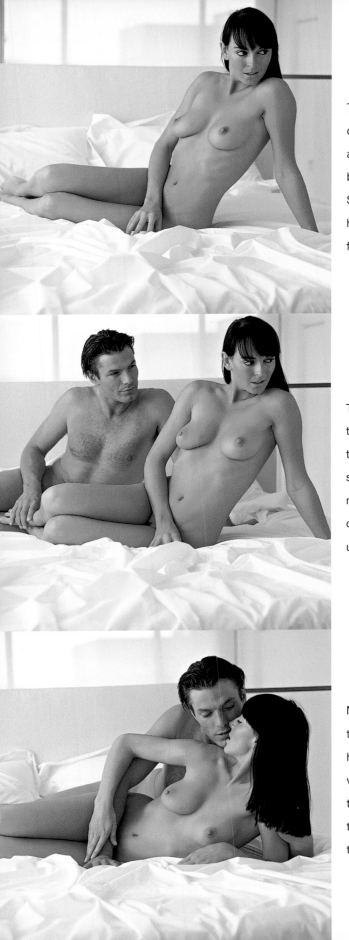

The woman sits down either on a bed or on a cushion on the floor. While keeping her knees and ankles together, she twists to one side so that her back is turned away from the entrance to the room. She supports herself with her hands and tilts her head, looking over her shoulder, as if she is waiting for the sound of her man approaching.

The man sits at her feet and tenderly caresses them, letting her know he has returned. The woman then turns her upper body round towards him, still supporting herself on her hands. Slowly, the man moves closer to her, and his caresses travel upwards over her legs, over her buttocks and along her back, until he can embrace her around her shoulders.

Now, he kisses her mouth full on and, as he does, the woman opens her legs so that he can penetrate her from behind while keeping his body protectively wrapped around hers. He thrusts in long, slow strokes that gradually dispel the sense of distance between the lovers, until they both reach a climax that restores the longed-for feeling of togetherness.

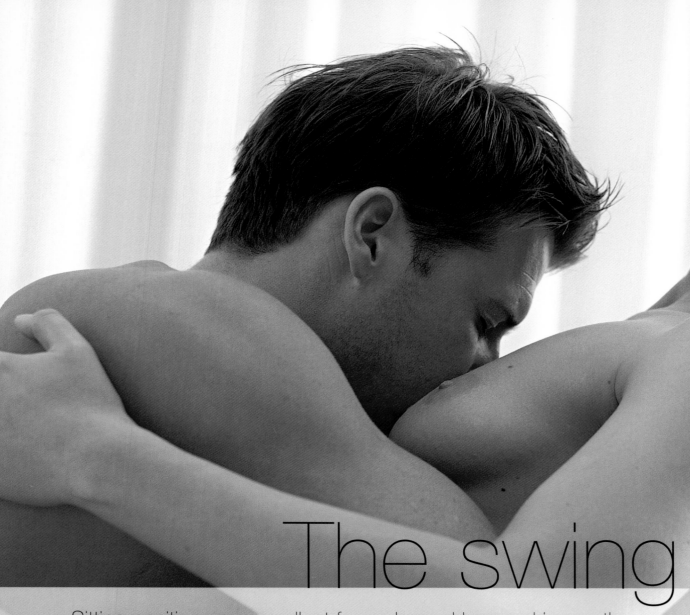

The swing

Sitting positions are excellent for prolonged love-making as they can be alternately energetic and restful. Maximize the pleasure by preparing the scene beforehand, making it comfortable for the long sex sessions to come. Partners can heighten intimacy by keeping eye contact while subtly varying their body movements. Many women find this a wonderful position for achieving orgasm while enjoying penetration.

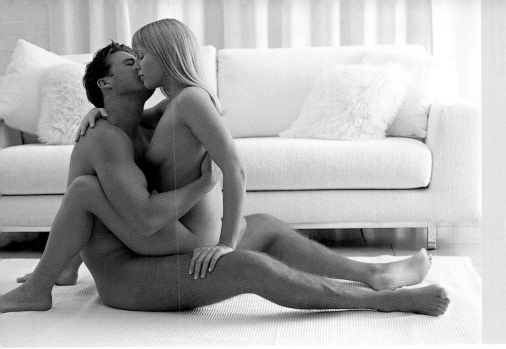

The couple sit close together, facing one another; the man's legs are open and the woman sits between them. She gently lifts her legs over his and tucks them around his back, resting her feet on the floor.

She drapes her arms around his neck, while he wraps his arms around her lower back. As she holds on, he guides her down on to his penis. Now, the lovers use the weight of their bodies to rock back and forth – just like a swing. Alternating more vigorous movements with gentler ones enhances the pleasurable sensations and prolongs the sex as well.

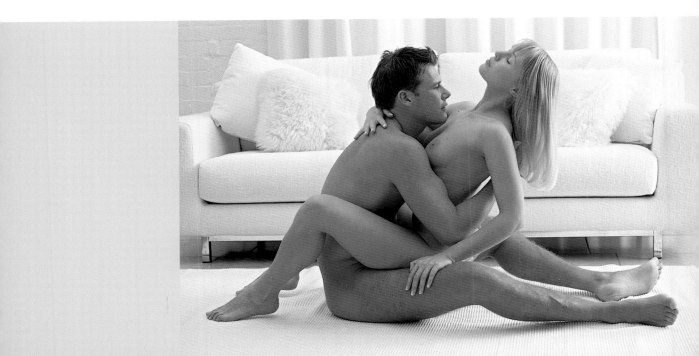

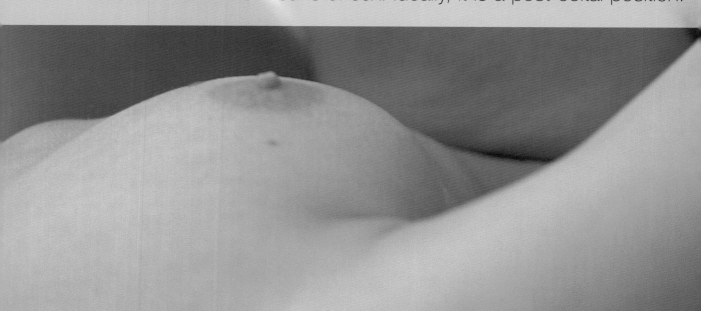

Namaste

Namaste is a Sanskrit word that literally means 'I bow to you';
its deeper meaning is 'my soul honours your soul'. In this tantric
posture the man honours his partner and, at the same time, the
divine feminine being that she embodies and with which his own
male divinity has been united in orgasm. It is both a way of saying
'thank you' and of aligning yourself with the sacred spark through
the means of sex. Ideally, it is a post-coital position.

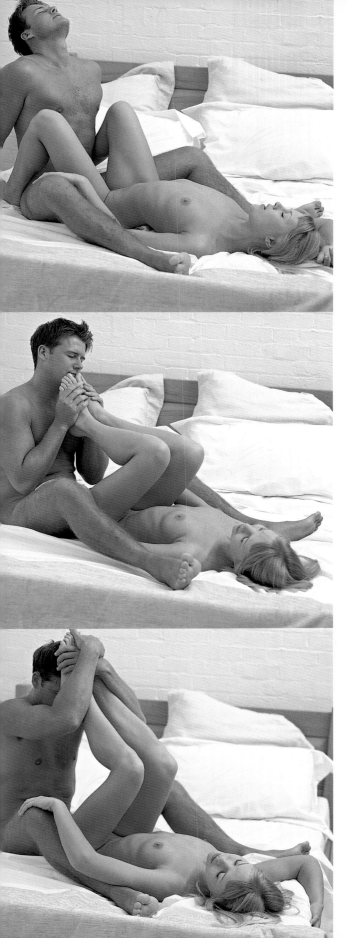

While sitting with his back straight the man parts his legs, bending his knees slightly. The woman lies on her back, her legs either side of his thighs, with her hips about level with his knees. At this point the man can penetrate the woman if he wishes, or he can just keep close bodily contact.

The man gently lifts her legs up towards his face, keeping them together with the knees bent, and places the soles of her feet against his mouth, so that he may kiss them.

He then holds her feet against his nose, followed by his eyes, his forehead and, finally, the crown of his head. In performing these movements, it is said that a man may fulfil all his desires.

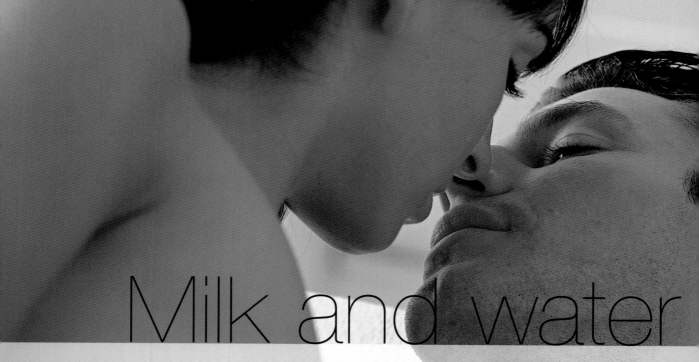

Milk and water

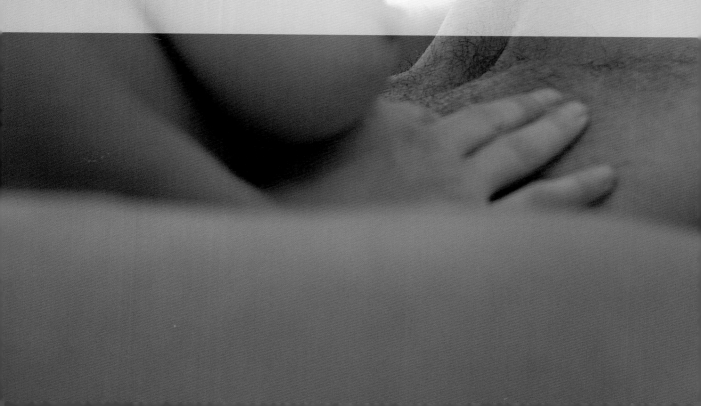

This embrace completes the cycle of intimate postures. It symbolizes a couple's desire to continue their togetherness and an unwillingness of each to let the other go. The couple in such an embrace could go on forever, as when one pauses the other can take up the rhythm again.

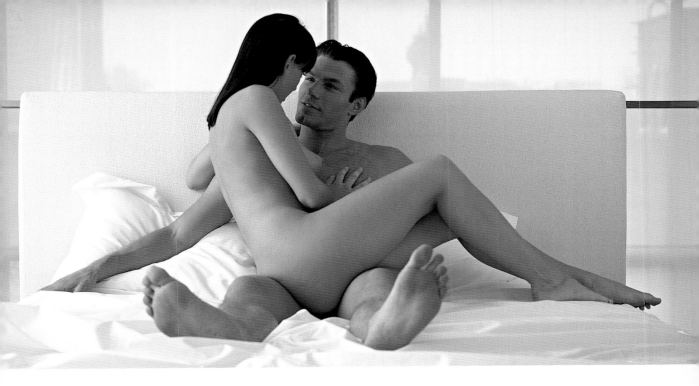

The woman lies across the man's lap, one arm thrown loosely around his shoulders. Then, she passionately kisses any part of his body she can reach and presses her body firmly against his from time to time, embracing and squeezing him with both arms and holding him to her as though she will never let him go.

The man hugs her with his arms around her waist and returns her kisses. He pulls her tightly to him whenever he feels the desire. In this way the lovers alternate active and passive roles in the embrace.

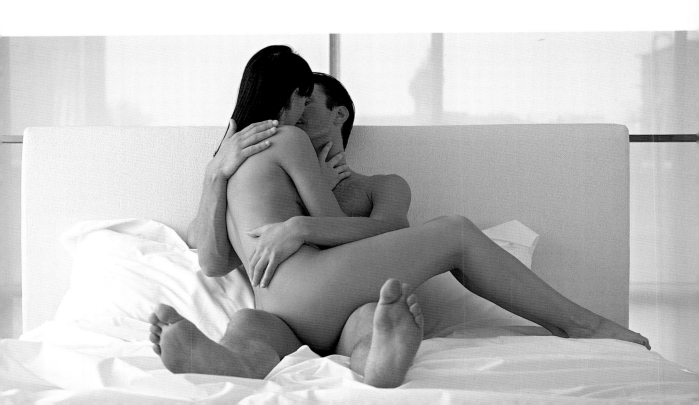

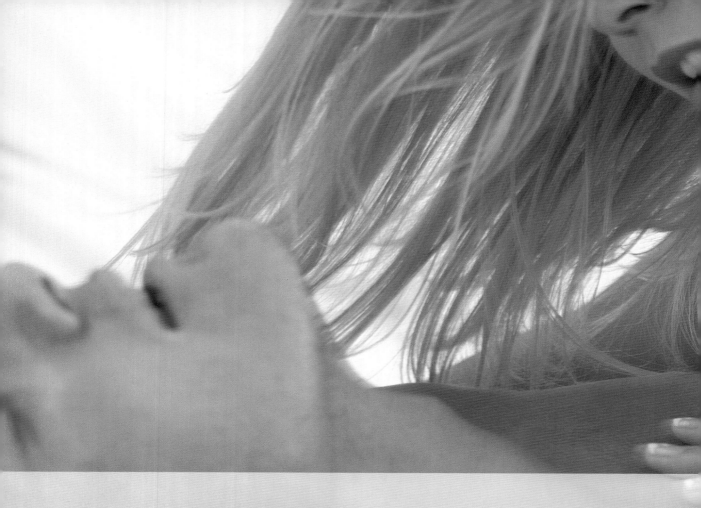

Passionate

Passion has depth; it may arise spontaneously or build up slowly. Passionate sex may be extremely physical or it may be slow and sensual. Surrender to your intense desires and see how the emotional bond between you and your partner grows stronger and stronger.

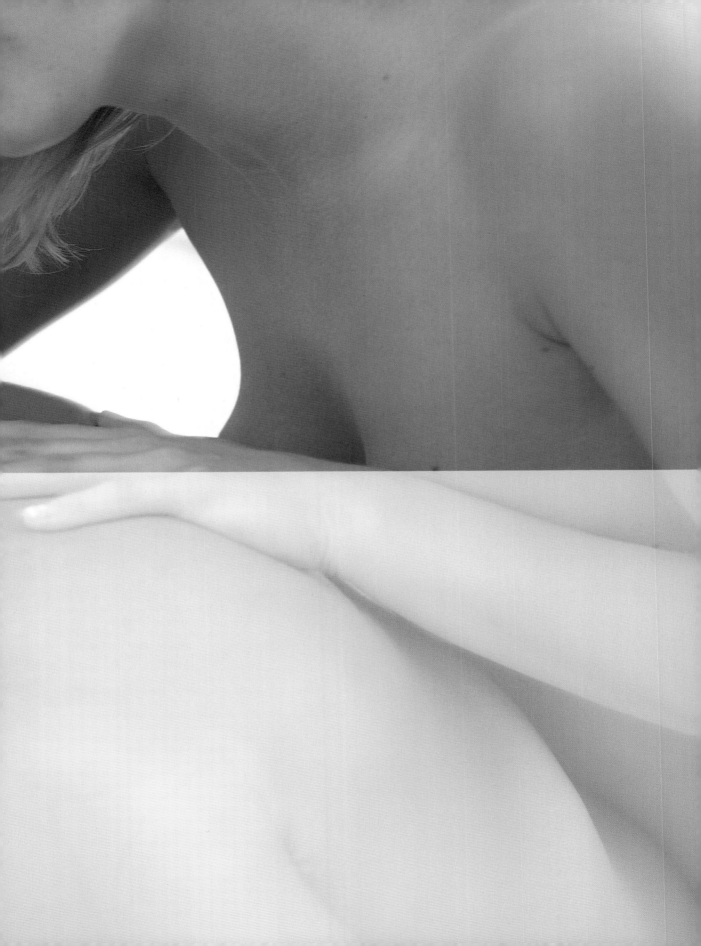

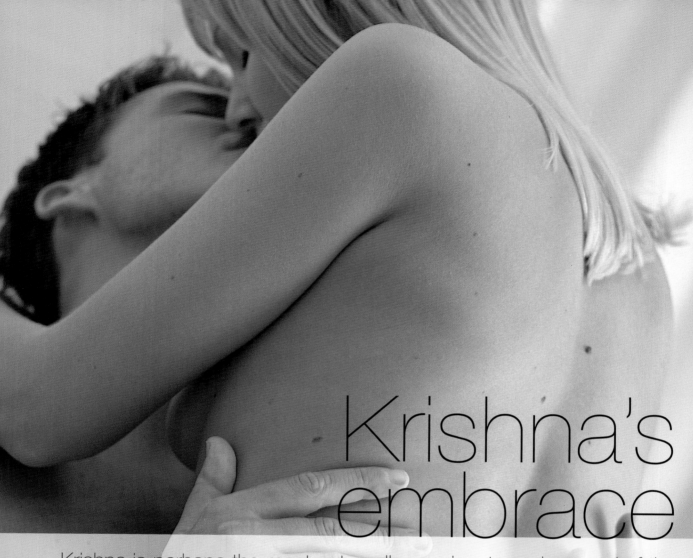

Krishna's embrace

Krishna is perhaps the most outwardly passionate and sensual of the Hindu deities. He knew something about spontaneity and that it is the essence of passion. There are moments when lovers look at each other and feel a sharp pang of desire. Act on it immediately, show the depth of your feelings and do not hold anything back.

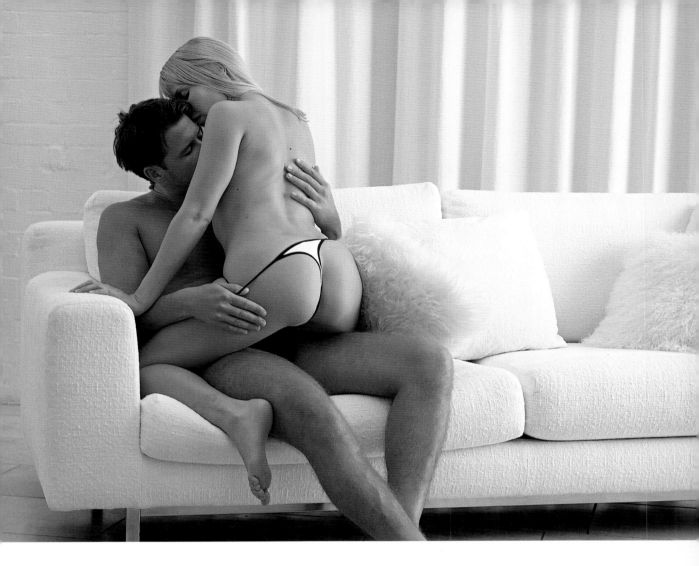

With the man sitting, the woman removes her shirt and bra, letting him see her breasts. She quickly straddles him and rubs her genitals against his thighs. As things hot up, she presses her breasts against him and, clasping him to her, passionately kisses his face, his eyes and his mouth.

In this embrace the woman initiates sex, throwing herself with passion at her lover.

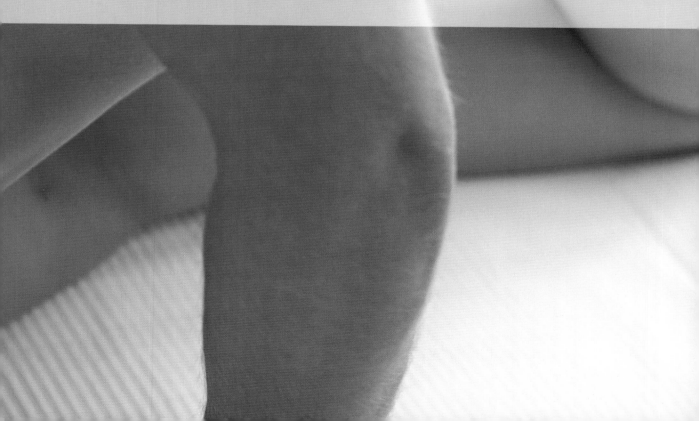

The tiger spring

The *Kama Sutra* and other Eastern texts often named positions after animals, and few animals have more sensual power of movement than the tiger. Some people call a passionate lover 'tiger' as an endearing way of drawing attention to their sexual appetite and their stamina.

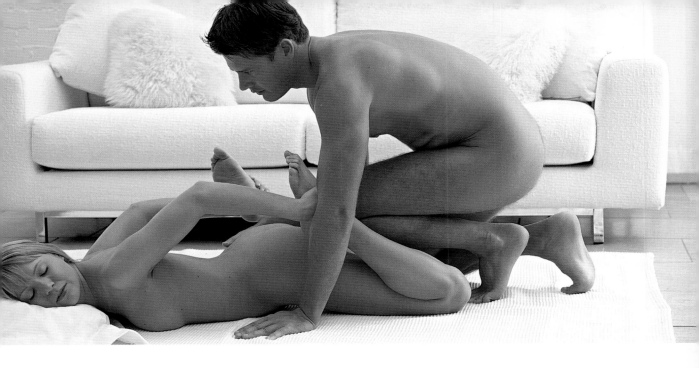

The woman lies flat on her belly, with her hips and breasts supported by soft cushions or a quilt on the floor and her head resting on a pillow. She bends her knees, raising her feet, and then reaches her arms back and grasps her ankles, holding on to them firmly.

The man kneels behind her and slips his thighs between hers, getting close enough to enter her. Leaning over her back, he can hold her by the waist or rest his hands on the ground as he thrusts deeply. Anyone with back problems should modify this pose to avoid any strain.

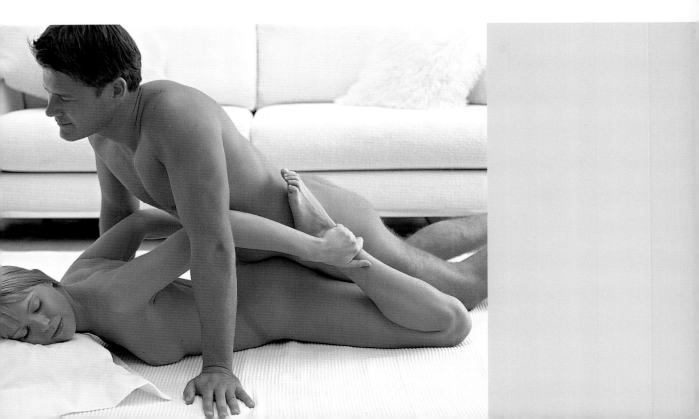

Archimedes' screw

This popular woman-on-top position fulfils many pleasurable functions. First, it permits the man to rest and to enjoy a more passive role. Second, he can watch the expression on his lover's face as well as her body moving above him, which in turn arouses him further. Third, the woman is in control of the rhythm and depth of penetration, which is exhilarating for her.

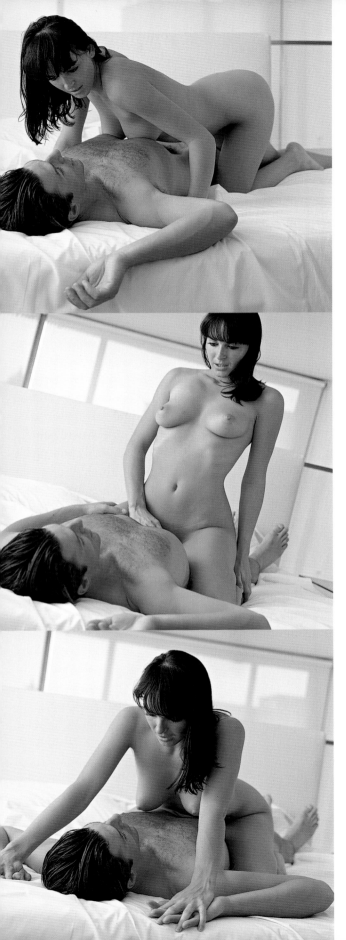

The man lies on his back on the bed, supporting his head with his hands if he wishes, while the woman sits astride his thighs. She can see her partner's responses to her movements clearly, and both can have frequent eye contact throughout.

Raising herself on her knees as much as necessary, she directs his penis inside her, and then slowly sinks back down to sit over his genitals. While in this pose, she can also stroke her own clitoris, giving her more control over her orgasms. Anyone who might feel inhibited about being observed so openly by a lover should bear in mind that men rarely think critically of women's bodies during sex and that they love to see their partner taking control and enjoying themselves.

Placing her hands either side of his head for support, she leans forward, keeping her belly away from his. The woman then dictates the motion and pace of the sex: moving up and down or in a circular motion, varying her movements and her rhythm as she pleases. In this way, both lovers can experience a variety of sensations.

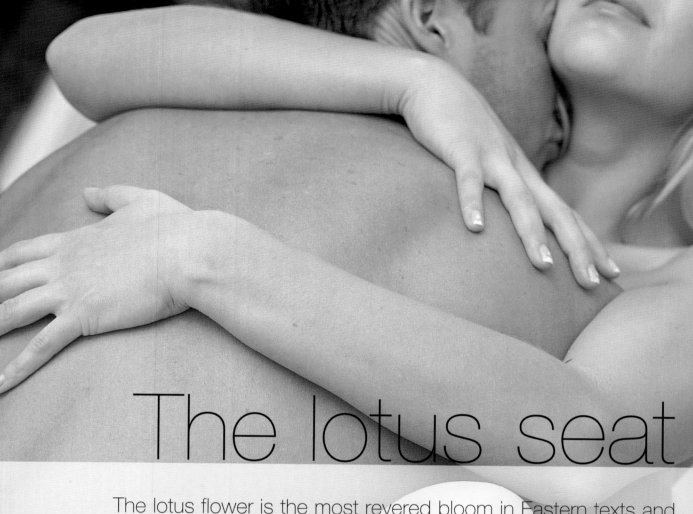

The lotus seat

The lotus flower is the most revered bloom in Eastern texts and the lotus seat, as a throne for a deity, is encountered throughout religious texts as well as in art and architecture. Less flexible couples may find this sitting posture tricky, but it can be easily adapted to use one leg over, similar to the half-lotus yoga *asana*.

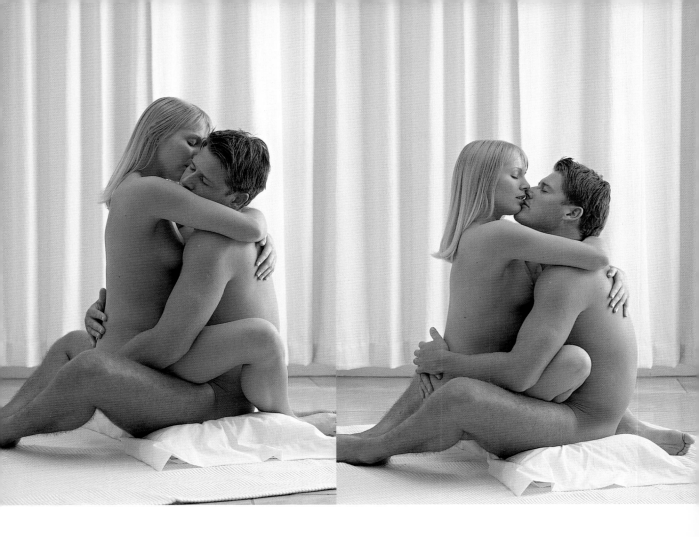

The man and woman stand facing one another and then sink down so that she sits in the gap between his legs. He then bends his legs loosely around her back. She then crosses her legs so that she assumes the lotus position, placing her left foot on his left thigh and her right foot on his right thigh. (An easier form of this posture is for the woman to put one leg around the man's waist and cross only one leg over.)

She keeps him close by wrapping her arms around his neck. He then pulls her closer and enters her, clasping her waist or holding her underneath her buttocks. Only the very supple will be able to achieve much movement in this posture, although the man can move the woman by supporting her buttocks and lifting her up and down.

Excellent for prolonged and sensual love making, experiment with this position to suit your suppleness.

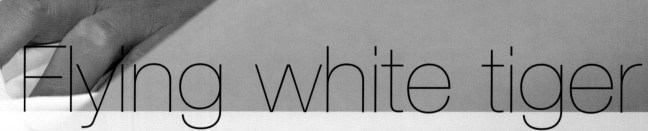

Flying white tiger

Rear-entry positions are extremely stimulating for men: they can penetrate more deeply while having more control over their thrusting. What's more, the view that they have of a woman in this posture is profoundly arousing for them. For the woman, the angle of penetration encourages stimulation of her G-spot. She can also determine the depth of penetration by altering the number of pillows or cushions she has underneath her belly and hips.

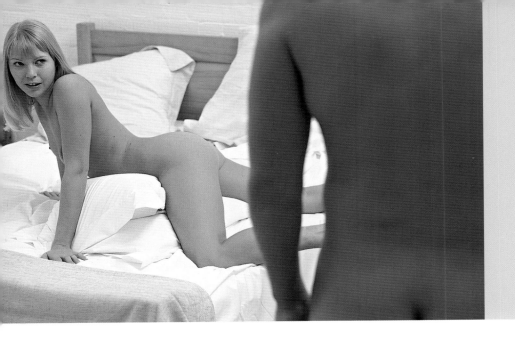

While the man watches her, the woman assumes a comfortable kneeling position, making sure that she can support herself in this posture for some time. She should take time arranging herself, aware that her lover is becoming aroused by watching her body movements. She may place cushions or pillows under her upper body, to lessen the load on her arms, and under her belly to determine the depth of penetration.

Highly aroused by now, the man kneels behind her and enters her immediately. He clasps her waist and pulls her towards him. A mixture of deep and shallow thrusting is ideal in this position and will prolong the enjoyment. Although the woman is unable to touch her clitoris in this posture, she may find that she can rub herself against the edge of one of the cushions to help her to climax.

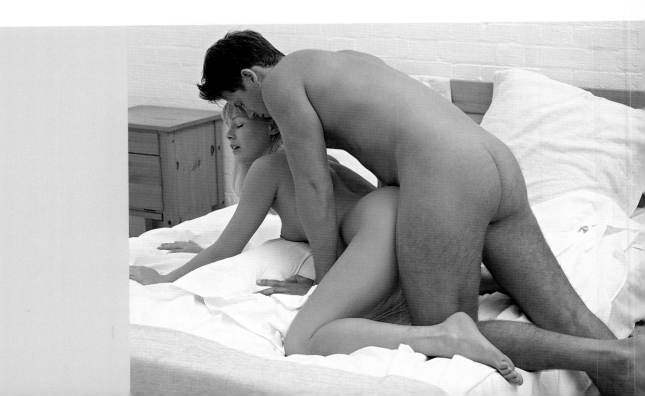

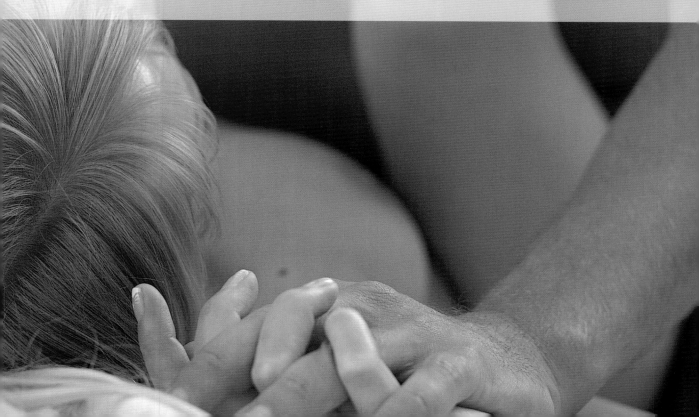

The swallow

Some face-to-face postures allow deep penetration, and many of them are variations on The Missionary (see page 12). There are two basic ways to vary this classic position: to raise the woman's buttocks on a cushion or to have the woman raise her legs, placing them on various parts of the man's body. The Swallow sees the woman adopt a position where her raised legs alter the shape of her vagina, thus making a very snug fit around her lover's penis.

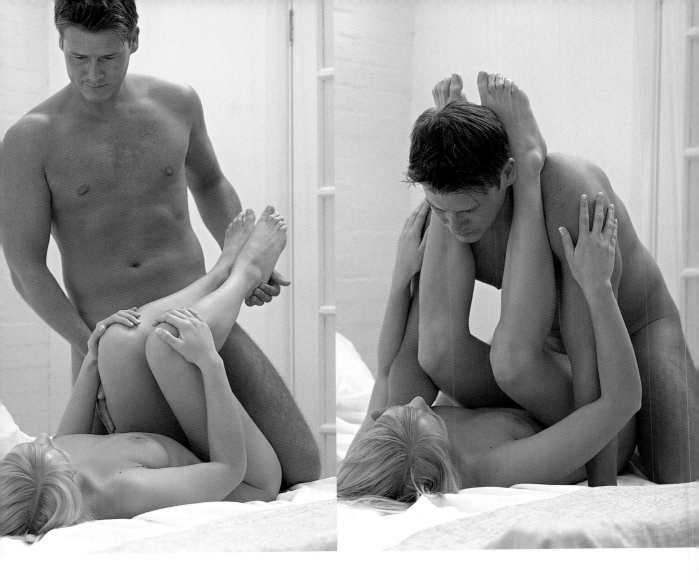

The woman lies on her back, with her head supported, and draws her knees right up to her chest, keeping her feet in the air. This bent-knee position allows her to display her genitals to the man, as well as making her vagina both shorter and tighter. The man approaches her in this highly arousing position and kneels down in front of her.

The woman moves her feet on to his shoulders, to give her support and prevent her leg muscles from becoming overtired. In this face-to-face position, he penetrates her while steadying himself on his hands. He takes control of the movement, varying the depth and rhythm of his thrusting so that both of them experience a range of sensations.

The Swallow is a very pleasurable position as it permits deep and tight penetration.

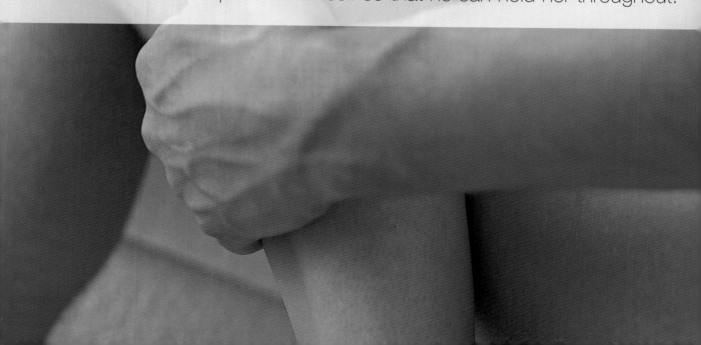

Swimming fishes

Many positions are helped by the strategic use of furniture, cushions or other objects around your home, and this is no exception. A low, comfortable sofa is best for this rear-entry position with a difference, the difference being that the woman is neither flat on her belly nor in a kneeling position. The man supports the weight of the woman's body, so he must take the time to position himself so that he can hold her throughout.

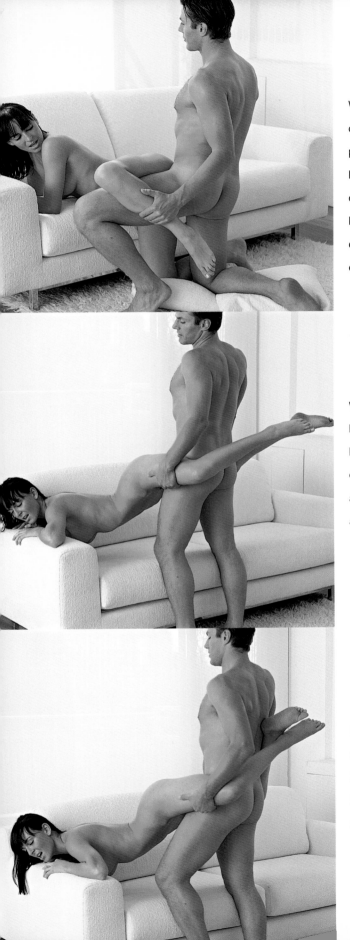

With the woman leaning slightly forwards on a low sofa or bed, the man approaches her from behind and positions his right knee on a floor cushion; his other knee remains raised at a right angle. The woman sits on his left knee, facing away from him, with her left knee facing forwards and her right knee on the floor, close to his right knee. She rests her elbows on the edge of the sofa or bed.

While the man holds on to her waist, she drops her body forward on to the sofa, letting it support most of her upper body weight. Now, he stands up and, as he does so, he slides his hands down the woman's thighs and lifts her legs up around his waist so that she is in a position where he can penetrate her.

Once he is inside her, she bends her legs at the knee and tucks them behind his back as he thrusts into her; this repositioning of her legs helps to keep her vagina tight around his penis for maximum stimulation for both lovers.

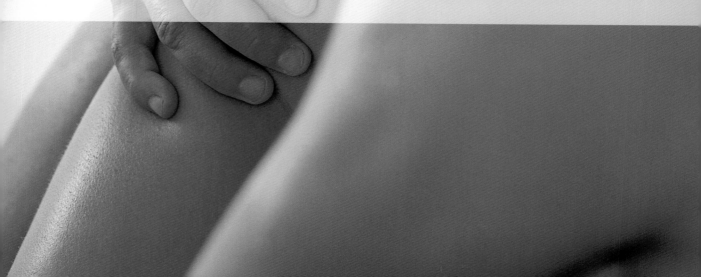

The camel's hump

This is a perfect posture for passionate sex and one that is very popular with men, as it offers a comfortable standing position where he can admire his partner's body. This hands-free position allows him to guide his penis inside her initially and then to stroke and fondle her breasts or her clitoris during thrusting.

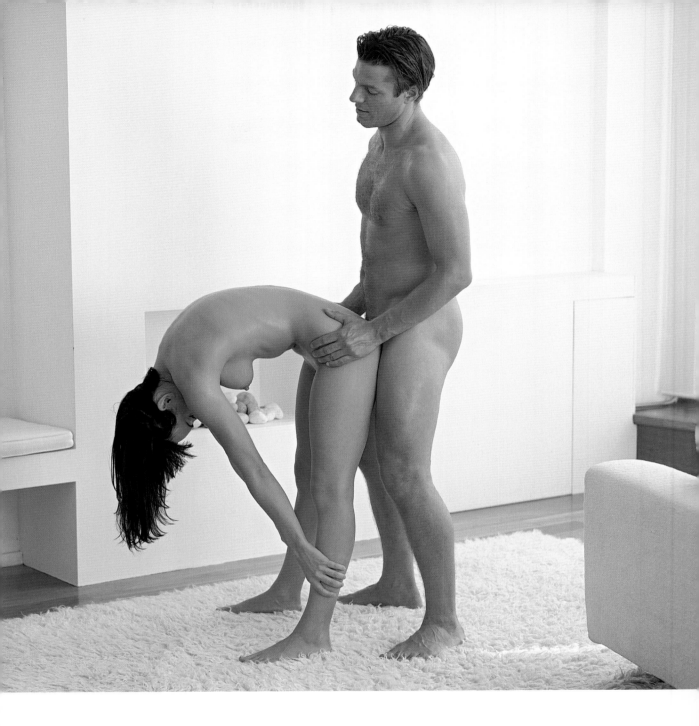

The woman stands with her back facing the man, then folds forwards from the waist until she is as close to touching her toes as possible. Unless she is incredibly supple and can reach the floor, it is a good idea to have a heap of floor cushions or items of furniture nearby (the edge of a sofa or armchair, for instance) so that she need only bend as far as is comfortable. The man admires her posture, comes to stand closely behind her and penetrates her, holding her steady by clasping her at the hips. In this position he has the exciting view of her genitals while also being able to watch and control the pace of his own hard thrusting movements.

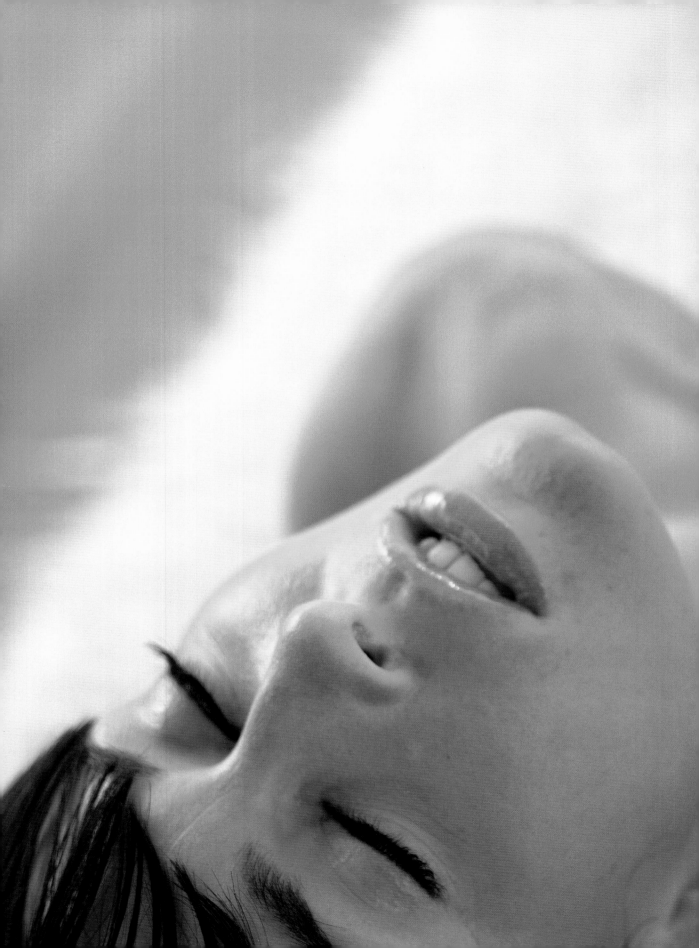

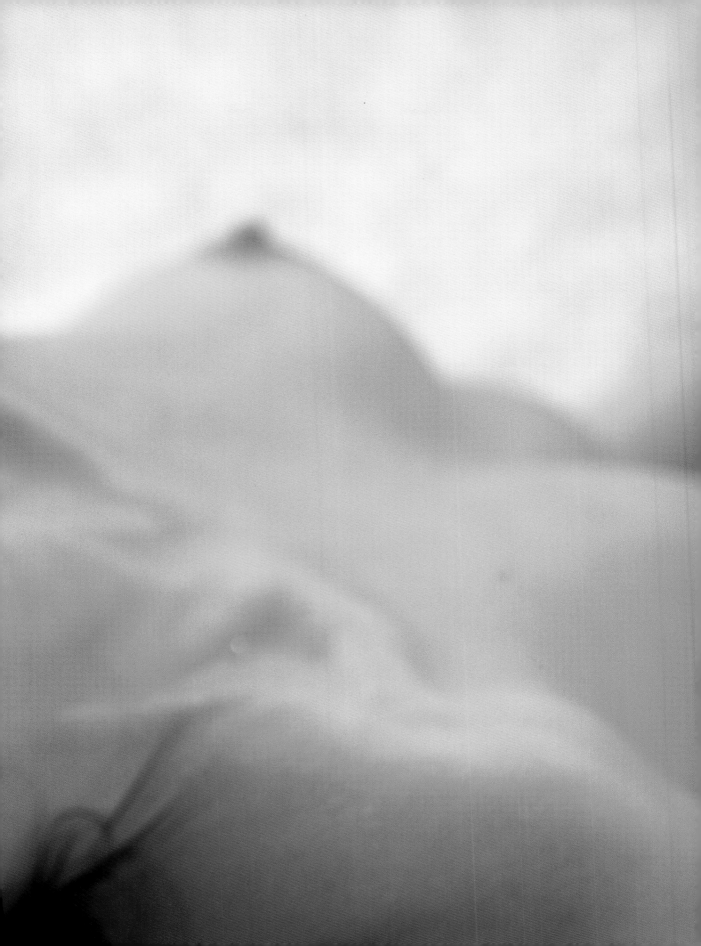

A pair of flying ducks

At times during sex you may want a private space where you can become absorbed in the sensations you are experiencing without having to communicate with your partner directly. This woman-on-top position, in which the woman faces away from the man, is one such posture. The man can relax and let her do the work, while admiring the movements of his lover on his erection.

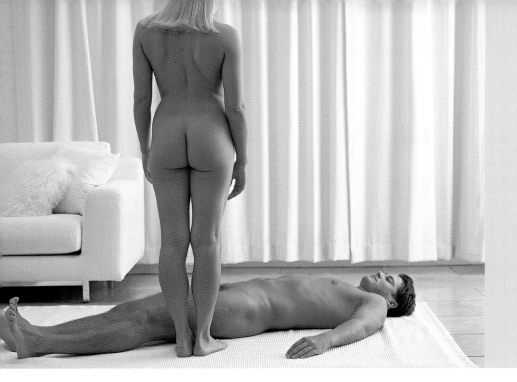

The man lies on his back with his legs stretched out straight and close together. It is best for the man to keep his body still in order to focus on his lover's movements and quilts on the floor or a firm bed provide the perfect platform for him to do this.

The woman kneels astride him, facing his feet. For those women feeling strong and supple, an alternative is to adopt a squatting position so as to try out a different angle of penetration. Whether kneeling or squatting, she sinks down on to his erect penis and uses various circular or up-and-down movements. During sex, she can use her free hands to stroke her clitoris and her breasts, while the man can play with her buttocks and back.

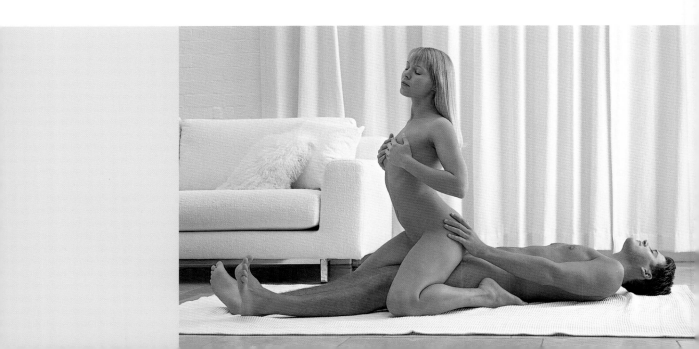

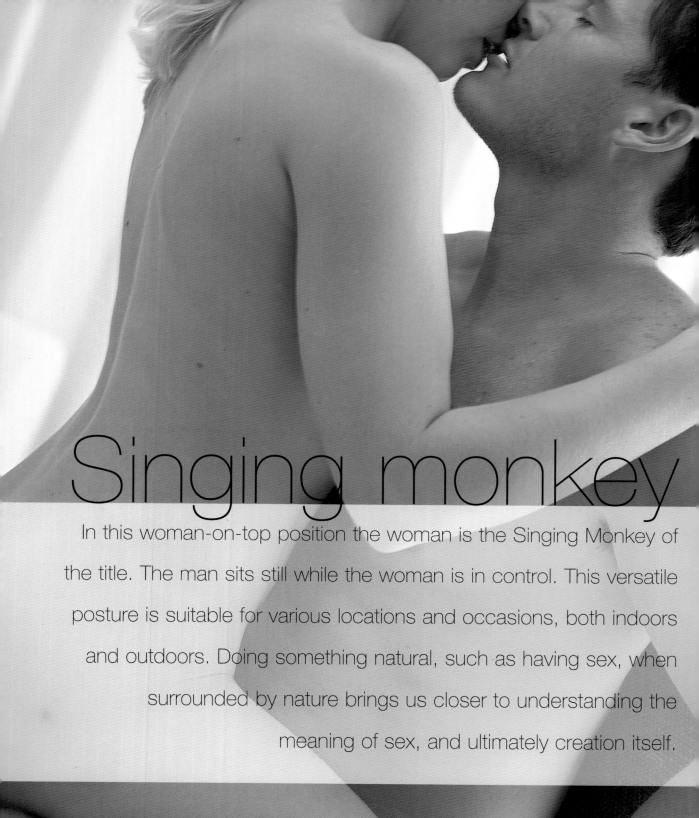

Singing monkey

In this woman-on-top position the woman is the Singing Monkey of the title. The man sits still while the woman is in control. This versatile posture is suitable for various locations and occasions, both indoors and outdoors. Doing something natural, such as having sex, when surrounded by nature brings us closer to understanding the meaning of sex, and ultimately creation itself.

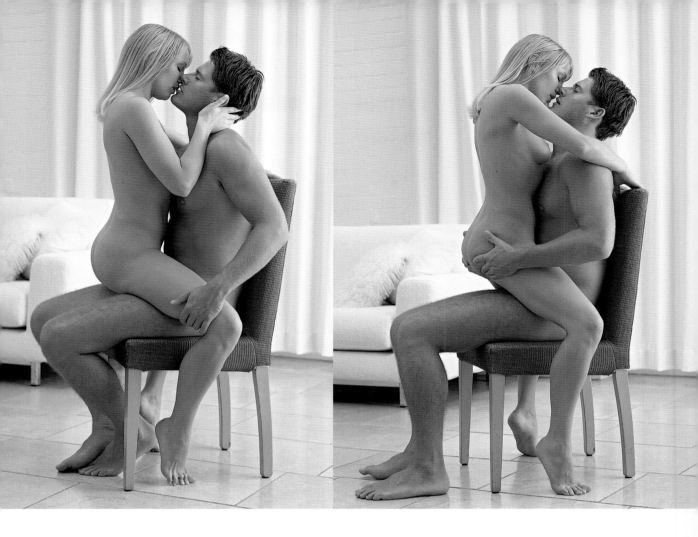

After grabbing a straight-backed chair, preferably with a cushioned seat, the man sits down and the woman quickly straddles his lap, facing him, and clasps her hands round the back of his neck. While keeping her feet on the floor, she lifts herself up and helps him to penetrate her.

The man fondles her buttocks with his hands and may control her movements on him. The couple can alternate between strong and gentle movements as well as taking turns to be the one in control. As an alternative, the woman can clasp her hands tightly behind his neck and lean back, perhaps balancing her feet on the bottom strut of the chair, if it has one. She would then have a greater range of movement and could circle her hips.

Try this position – indoors or outdoors – when you fancy a change from the bedroom.

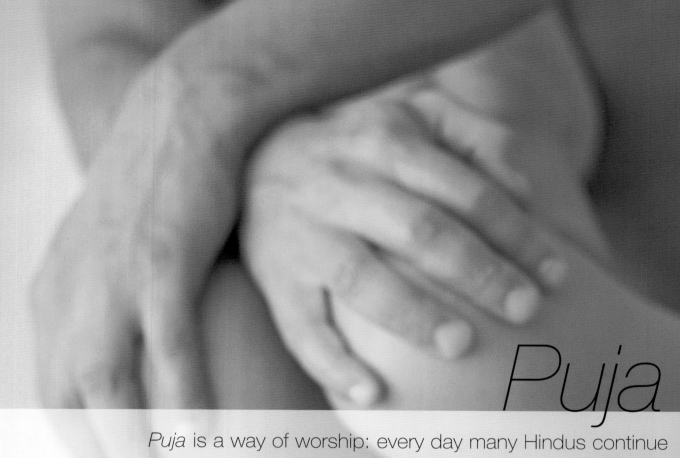

Puja

Puja is a way of worship: every day many Hindus continue to make an offering of flowers before an altar of the gods, light the incense and make a prayer. Sex is also a form of *puja*. In this posture there is a closed circuit of energy, one in which the male and female energies form a whole. In the tantric texts, it is this wholeness that brings us to enlightenment.

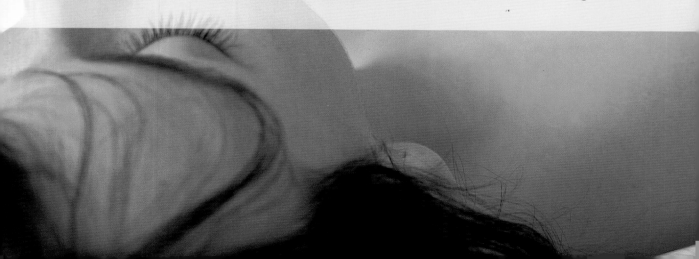

In this face-to-face position, the woman lies relaxed on her back and the man, kneeling to face her, helps her to raise her knees towards her chest. Once she is comfortable, he slides his knees so that they are either side of her hips and places her feet against his chest so that her legs are supported.

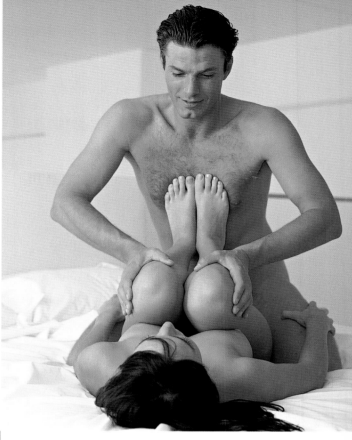

When he enters her, he takes charge of the movement. He holds her knees together by crossing his arms over the top of them, which helps him to thrust more energetically. While her knees are held together, her vagina can grip him more tightly and heighten this pleasurable experience for both of them.

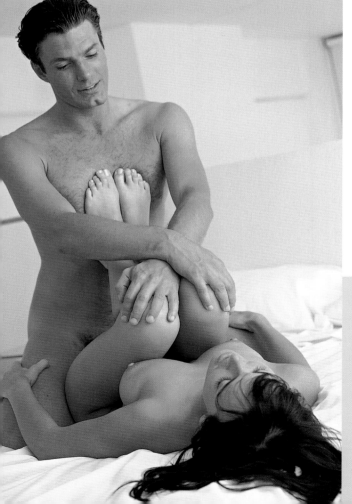

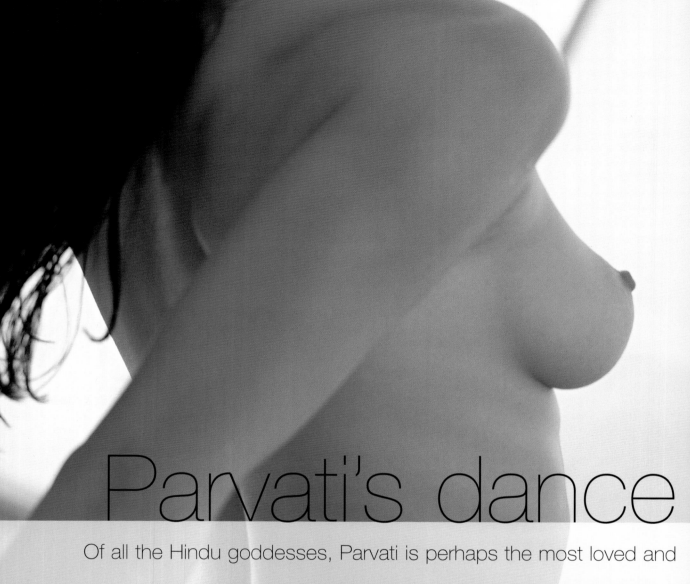

Parvati's dance

Of all the Hindu goddesses, Parvati is perhaps the most loved and the most giving of her love. Parvati represents a celebration of womanhood. Considered to be the epitome of sensual beauty, she represents both the physical and the spiritual. This woman-on-top position allows real expression of passion and a wonderful closeness.

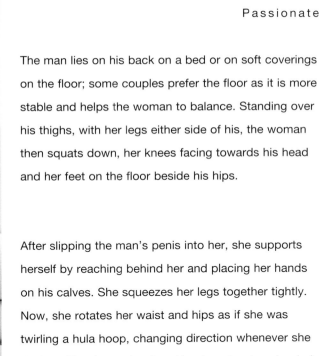

The man lies on his back on a bed or on soft coverings on the floor; some couples prefer the floor as it is more stable and helps the woman to balance. Standing over his thighs, with her legs either side of his, the woman then squats down, her knees facing towards his head and her feet on the floor beside his hips.

After slipping the man's penis into her, she supports herself by reaching behind her and placing her hands on his calves. She squeezes her legs together tightly. Now, she rotates her waist and hips as if she was twirling a hula hoop, changing direction whenever she desires. She throws her head back and swings her hair as if she has just emerged from a watery dip and is shaking off the excess droplets. If the woman finds it hard to balance while squatting, she should hold her lover's hands, interlacing her fingers with his and pressing her palms against his to steady her.

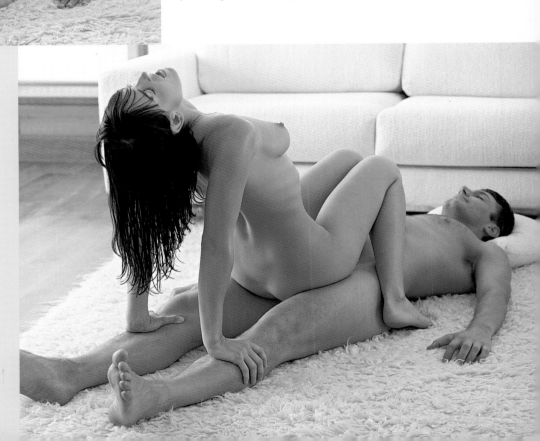

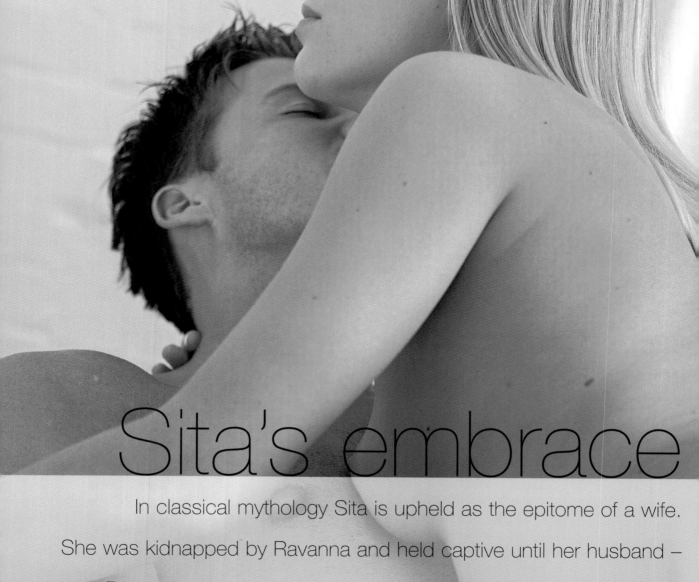

Sita's embrace

In classical mythology Sita is upheld as the epitome of a wife. She was kidnapped by Ravanna and held captive until her husband – Rama – rescued her. Ravanna had tried endlessly to force her to have sex with him but she had always resisted. Once home, she walked through a fire to demonstrate her absolute fidelity.

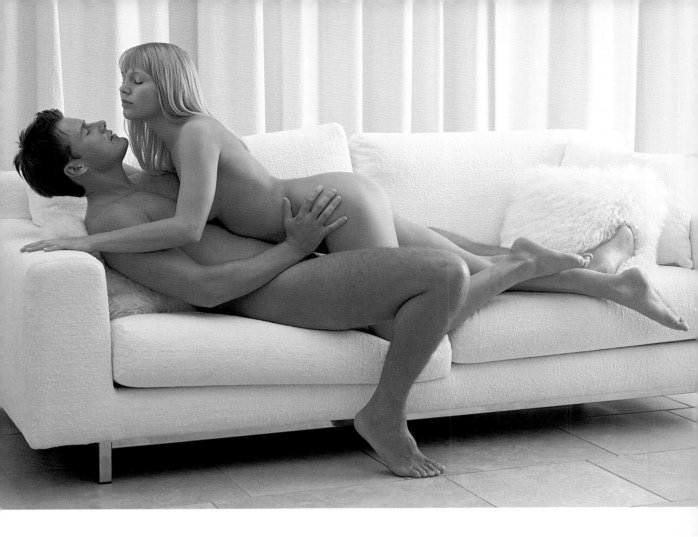

This embrace allows the woman to show her devotion to her lover. With the man lying or sitting on a sofa or chair, the woman clasps him to her and rubs her breasts feverishly against his chest before moving over the rest of his body as she wishes. She lets him feel the weight of her breasts, especially as she lies over his chest.

If she is clothed for this embrace, she should rip off her clothes to expose her breasts – no other part of her is important.

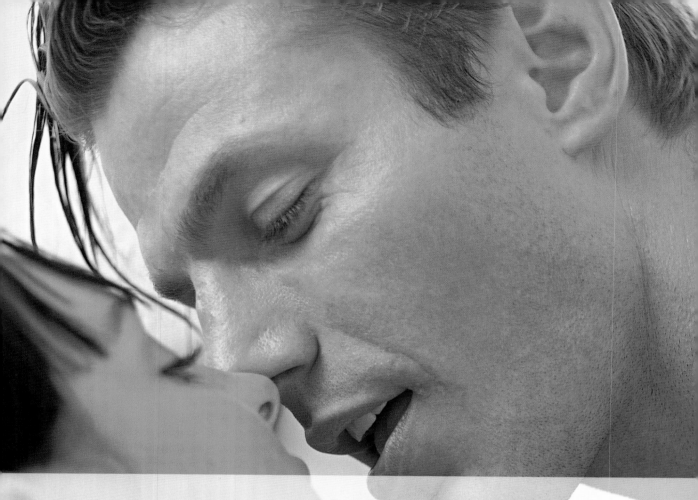

Energetic

Energetic sex usually arises in moments of heightened desire when we want instant fulfilment. Giving way to this urge is a way of refreshing your relationship and keeping it constantly renewed. There is a subtle difference between energetic and passionate sex: while passionate sex may be slow and sensuous, energetic sex is, by definition, 'fast sex' rather than slow.

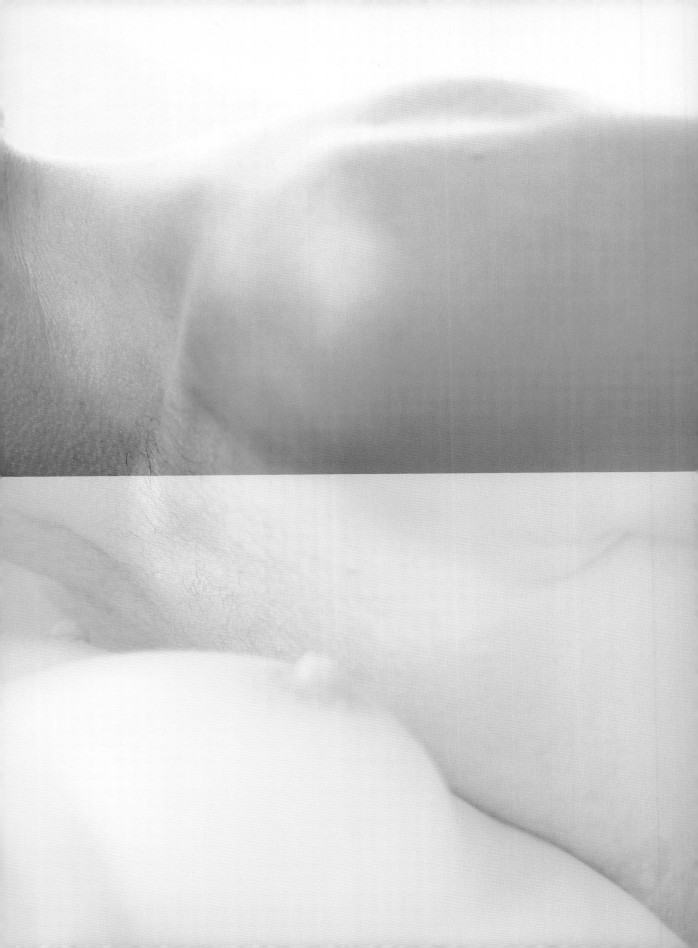

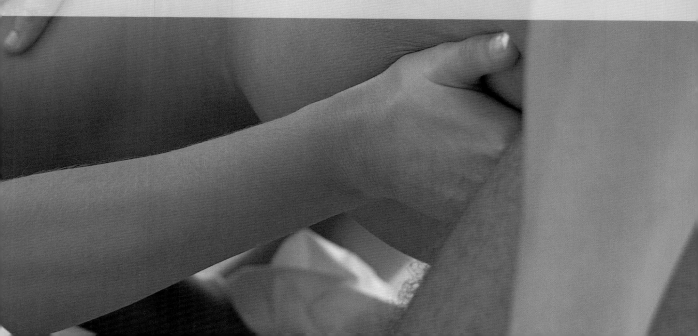

The open flower

This simple position is a variation on The Missionary (see page 12). However, it is energetic in the sense that it is a fairly physical pose, particularly for the woman, who must keep her pelvis raised. In this position, her legs are splayed, thus widening the vagina and allowing the man easier and faster entry. Her raised buttocks also permit deeper penetration by the man, helping to provide the strong sensations that are desired in fast sex.

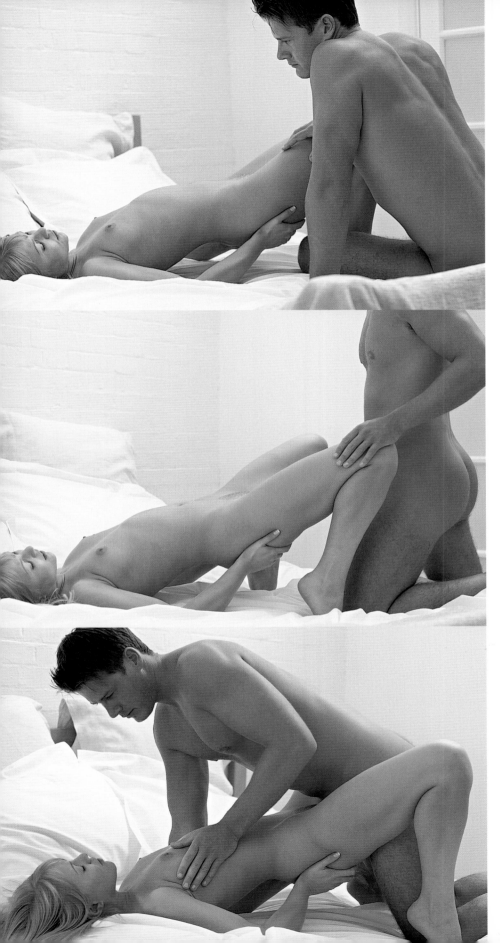

With the man sitting beside her, the woman lies on her back and tilts her pelvis upwards by supporting her buttocks on her hands.

Parting her legs, she bends her knees up and brings her heels back as far as she can towards her hips, keeping her pelvis raised off the bed.

The man takes up his position, kneeling between her legs, and penetrates her. He leans forward, supporting his weight on one hand while using the other to fondle her breasts.

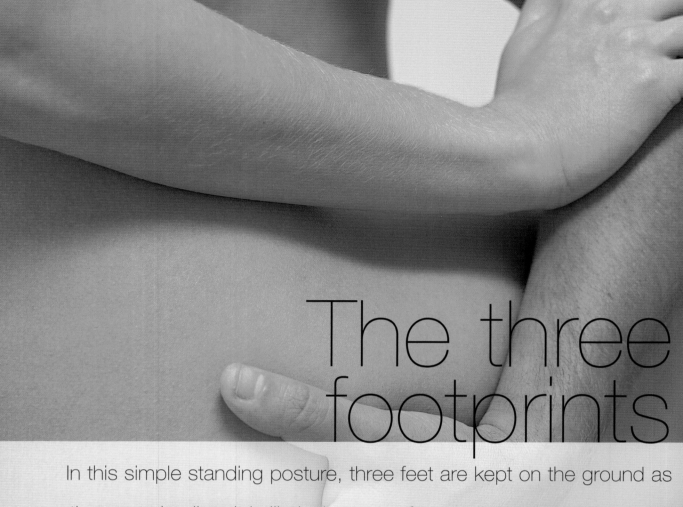

The three footprints

In this simple standing posture, three feet are kept on the ground as the name implies. It is likely that one of you will need some support, if only so that you can move without falling over. If there is a big height difference between you, use stairs to even things up; alternatively, telephone directories or a footstool may also work.

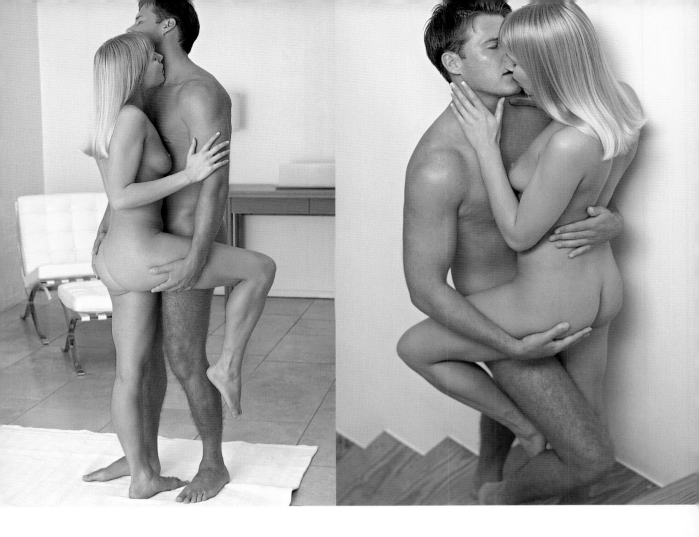

The man and woman stand facing each other, bodies touching. While keeping both feet on the ground, he supports her while she lifts one of her legs and, depending on height difference, wraps it around either his waist or his upper thigh. With her leg raised he now enters her. He offers her further support by placing one hand under her buttock and the other under the thigh of her raised leg.

Sometimes you won't want to wait until you reach the bedroom. If so, the stairs are an ideal location for sex in this posture, especially if the man is much taller than the woman.

Standing postures imply instant gratification, be it in a hallway or kitchen, a quiet alley or even against a tree.

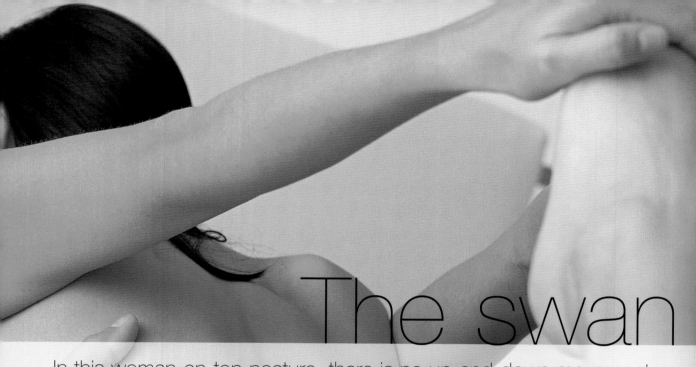

The swan

In this woman-on-top posture, there is no up-and-down movement on the penis. Rather, the pleasure of the posture relies on the ability of the woman to move her hips vigorously in circular or side-to-side motions. It is probably a posture that cannot be sustained for long, but it offers a highly unique experience and might be used for short bursts as a means of prolonging intercourse while varying the sensations.

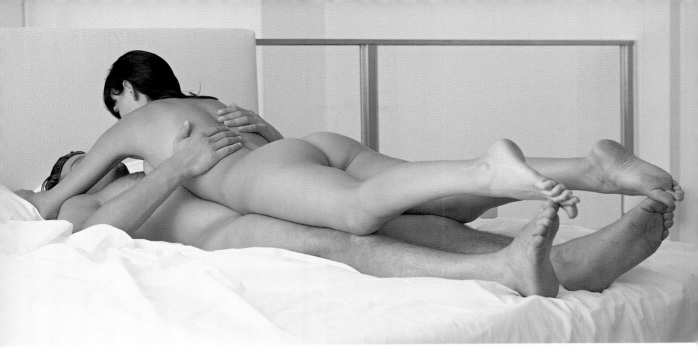

The man lies on his back on the bed with his legs together. The woman sits astride him, facing him, and guides his penis inside her. She then lowers her upper body on to his while bringing her legs up to lie along his thighs, so that she is lying along his entire length.

She now raises her lower legs, bringing her feet towards her buttocks, and clasps her feet or ankles with her hands. In this position she rocks her hips vigorously from side to side, or in a circular motion if she can, until both partners climax.

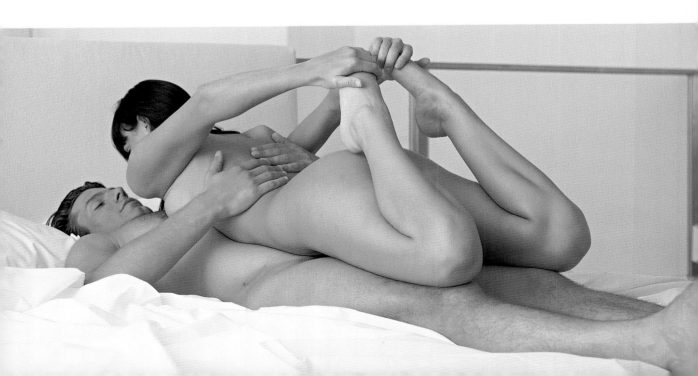

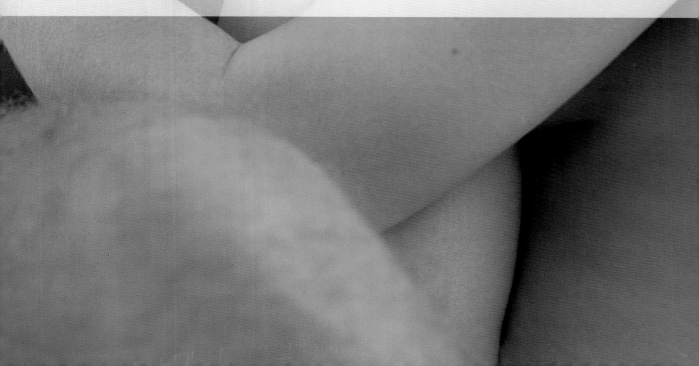

Two cobras entwined

The cobra is an important symbol in Hindu mythology. It represents power and fertility and is associated with the gods Shiva and Vishnu. Cobras are also thought to live in pairs, hence the name of this position. Although this sitting posture is one of the more difficult ones to achieve, it can be easily adapted to suit individual abilities.

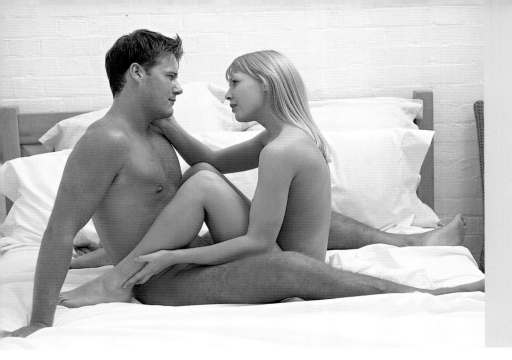

The woman sits upright (against a bed or sofa if she wants to support her back), and her lover sits facing her, spreading his legs either side of her hips. She draws her knees up towards her and places her hands under her calves, ready to lift up her legs.

Her partner enters her, holding her tightly to him by clasping his hands around the back of her neck. They now rock their bodies back and forth. The woman's vagina is tight in this posture and, while neither partner may achieve orgasm in this position, it is one that can take them towards a climax.

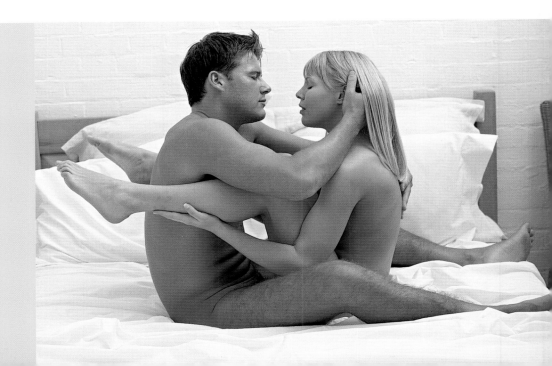

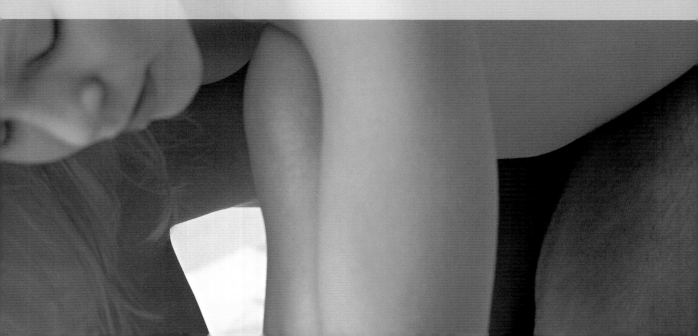

The plough

This position is extremely pleasurable for both lovers as it offers the possibility of many forms of stimulation. Before entry, the man can tenderly kiss the woman's neck and shoulders, fondle her breasts, and stimulate both her G-spot and clitoris simultaneously. Meanwhile, he can achieve deep penetration, thrust harder and, at the same time, use the visual stimulation of the rear-entry view to bring him to a climax.

While keeping his legs together, the man kneels and the woman sits astride his lap, facing away from him. The floor is the ideal place to perform this but make sure there are plenty of cushions to protect the man's knees. While in this posture he can caress her breasts and play with her clitoris, even bringing her to orgasm; he can also pepper her neck and shoulders with kisses.

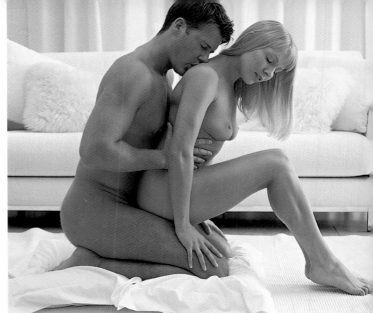

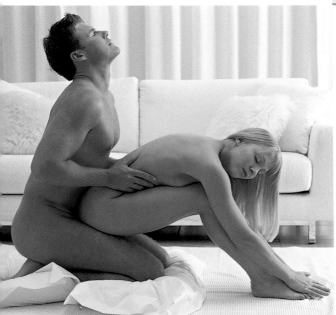

She then bends forward at the waist until she is in a prayer-like position, supporting herself on her hands and forearms. If it is more comfortable she can lean on a pile of pillows so she can rest her head. Now he enters her.

Finally, she stretches both of her legs back, one at a time, so that they extend out behind him. She rests her forearms on the ground for balance. Holding her by the hips or thighs, he thrusts deep inside her.

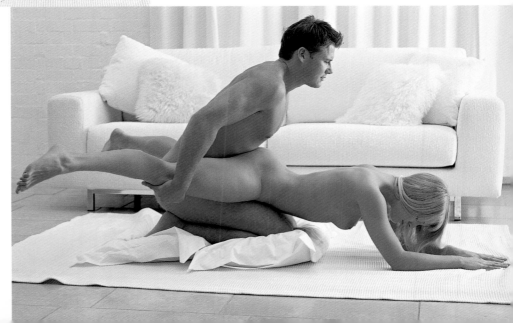

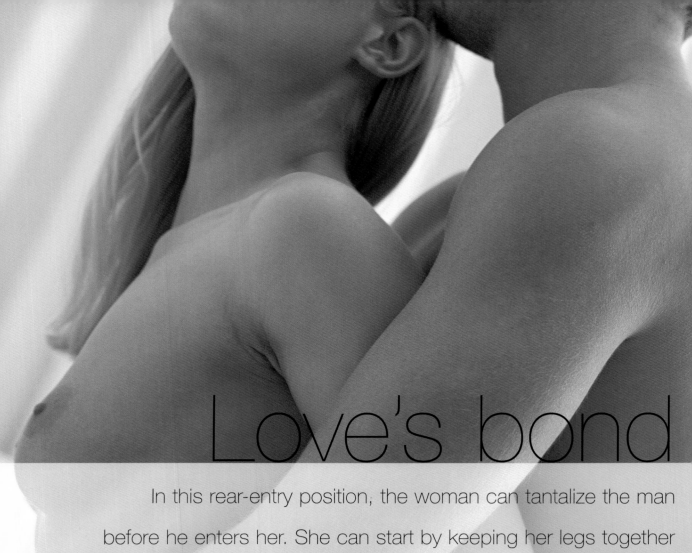

Love's bond

In this rear-entry position, the woman can tantalize the man
before he enters her. She can start by keeping her legs together
exposing little of her genitals, then part them slightly and wiggle
her hips. She can tease him by leaning away from him and
then back, only adopting the entry position with her legs fully
spread when she knows he can't wait any longer.

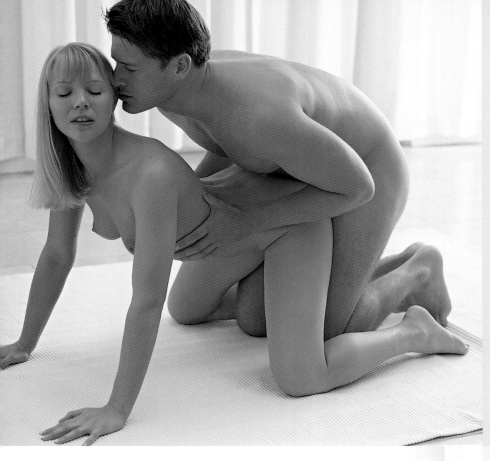

The woman takes up a kneeling position in front of the man, supporting herself on her hands, initially with her arms straight. She then arranges her legs so that he has a clear view of her vulva. Seeing her vulva clearly exposed in this rear-entry position is highly arousing for him. He drops to his knees behind her and thrusts his penis inside her, grabbing her around the waist.

Finally, she slips her arms around his elbows. He pulls her body up towards him and clasps her around her belly. (If this is uncomfortable, pile cushions up to offer support underneath her.) In this entwined position they can climax together.

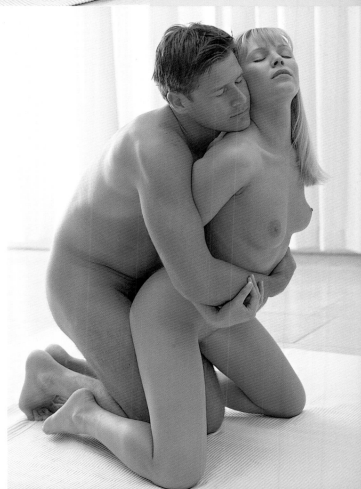

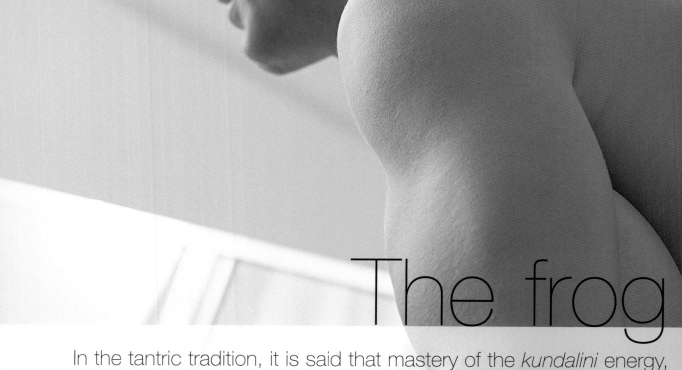

The frog

In the tantric tradition, it is said that mastery of the *kundalini* energy, which lies coiled like a serpent at the base of the spine, leads to the ability to jump like a frog. In the West, kissing frogs allegedly turns them into princes – here we hope you are already kissing your prince.

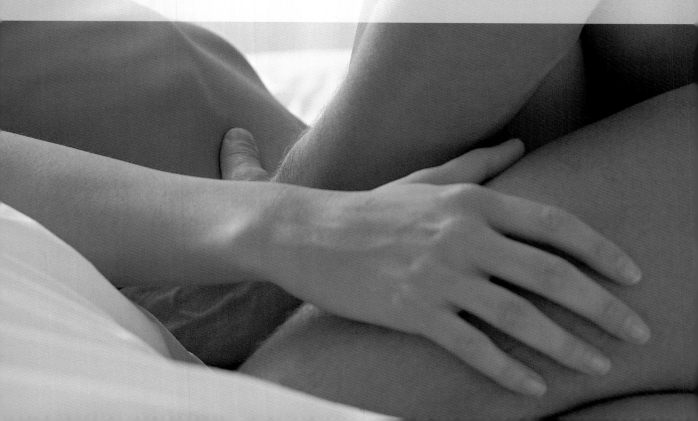

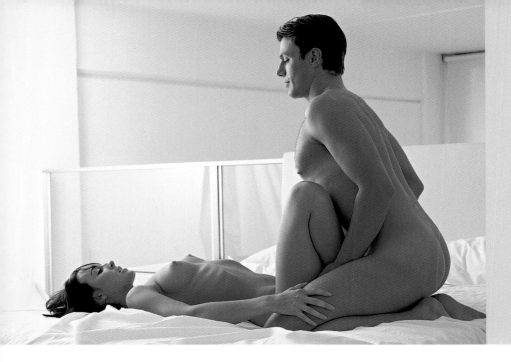

After falling hurriedly on to a bed, the woman lies on her back while the man kneels in front of her and lifts her legs so they bend at the knees. Gently he pushes her feet back towards her buttocks. Ideally, her heels should touch her buttocks, but this may be difficult; push them back only as far as is comfortable.

He eases himself into position between her legs and enters her. He holds her knees in place by gripping them under his armpits. There is a final manoeuvre to this position, which you should attempt only if you are feeling agile: at the moment of ejaculation, he places his hands under her back and pulls her up towards him.

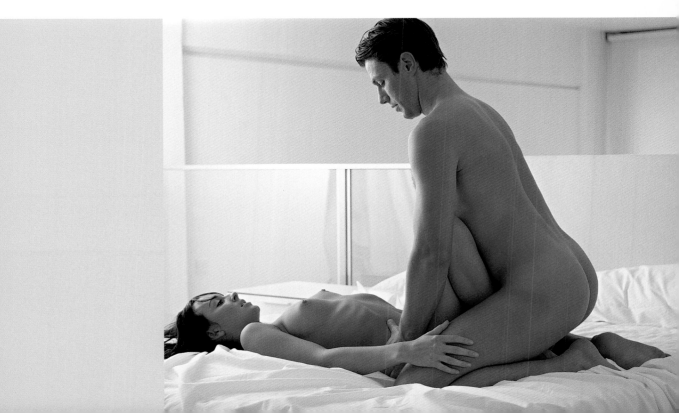

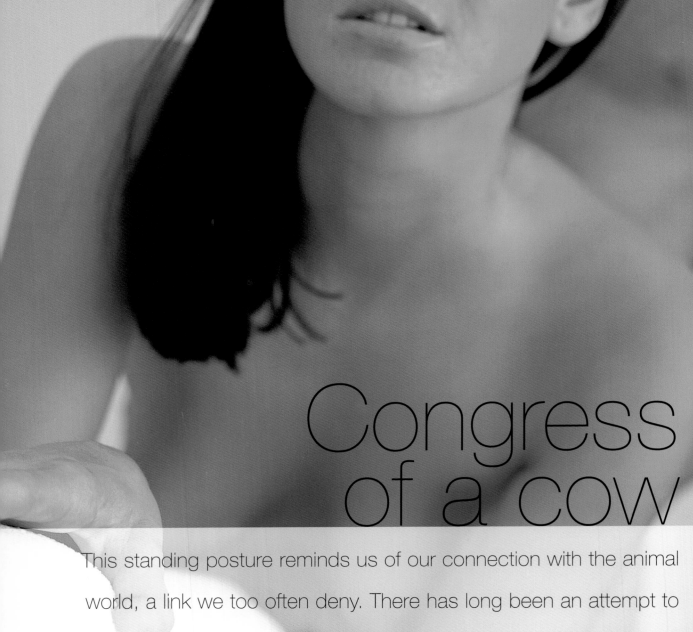

Congress
of a cow

This standing posture reminds us of our connection with the animal world, a link we too often deny. There has long been an attempt to distance ourselves from pleasures of the flesh, based on the idea that they remove us from what is sacred and divine. In fact, the opposite is true: through pleasure we come closer to knowing what is truly divine.

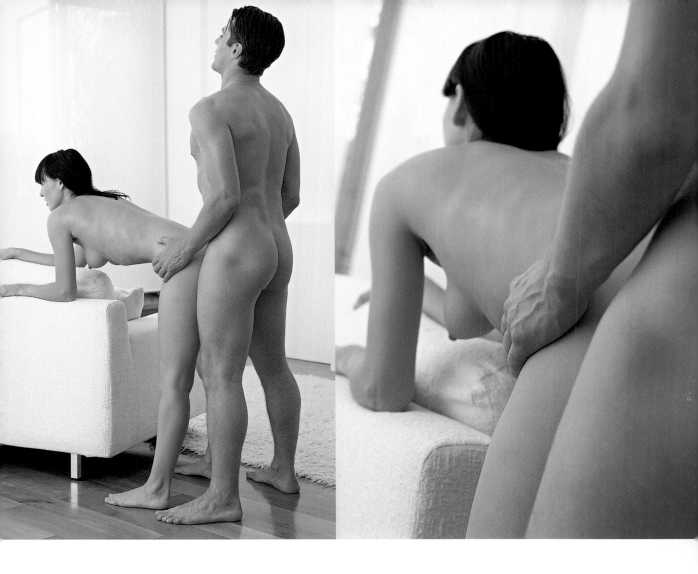

The woman stands in front of the man, facing away from him. She folds forward from her waist and bends to touch the floor, or leans on a piece of furniture, and supports herself with her hands. (The woman should bend over only as far as is comfortable and use any available furniture – bed, sofa, table, chair – for support.)

The man approaches her from behind as she stands in this highly arousing position and, as it says in the *Kama Sutra*, 'mounts her like a bull', clasping her tightly around the waist. As she is supported, she can join in by moving her hips against his thrusts to enhance both their pleasure.

This position indicates a sense of urgency: of fast and much-desired intercourse.

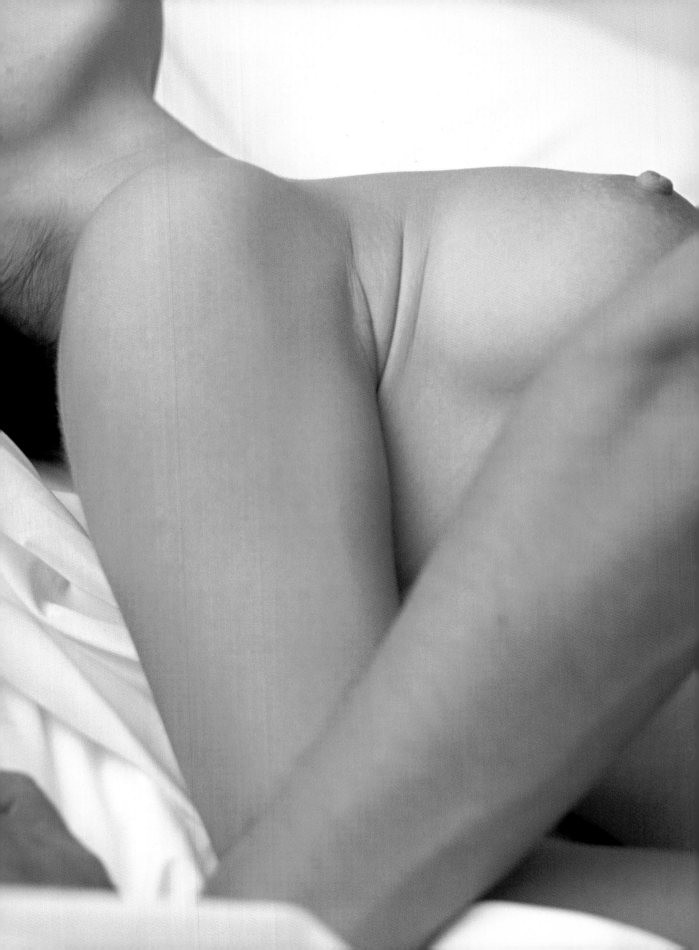

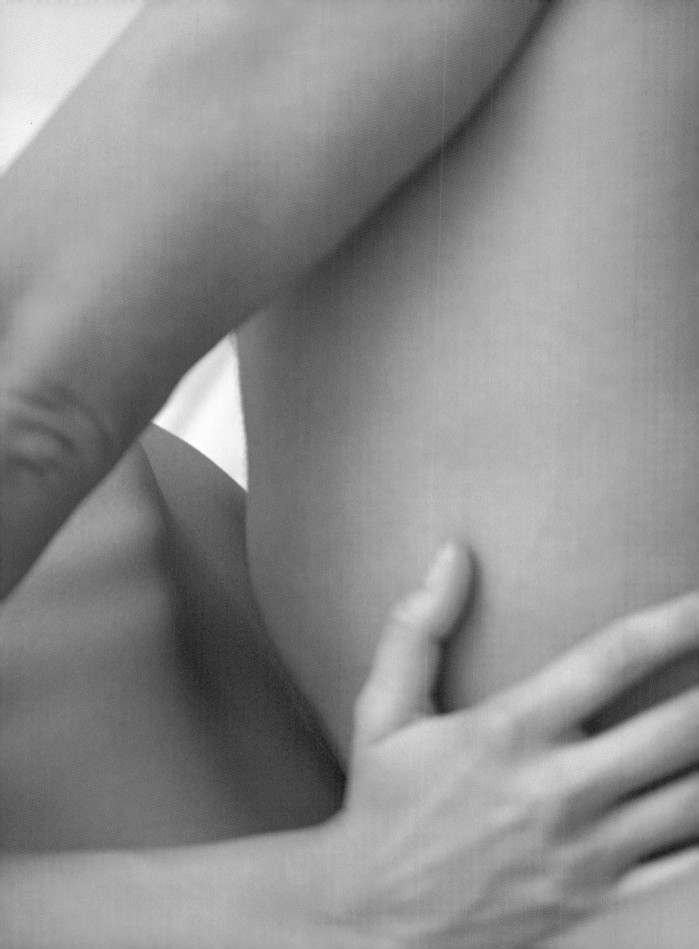

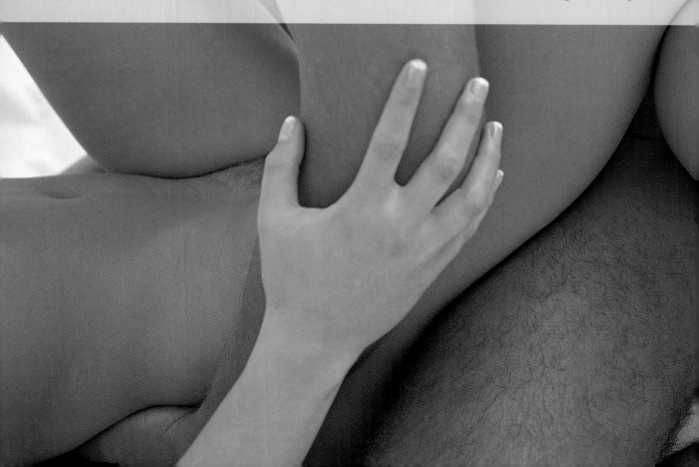

Splitting the bamboo

Although the woman lies on her back in this position she is the one in control of movement; the man remains still throughout. Many men find it extremely pleasurable when women actively take charge of sex. To relinquish control in this way relieves the man of any burden that he is somehow solely responsible for creating sexual pleasure. This is an ideal position for the woman who can create an energetic rhythm.

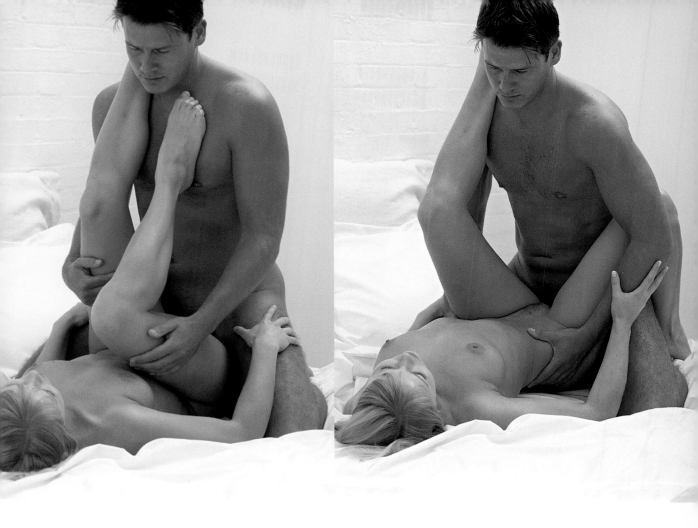

Once the woman is lying down on her back on the bed or on cushions on the floor, the man drops to his knees and kneels facing her. She stretches out one leg and places it over the man's shoulder. She bends her other leg back towards her chest and carefully positions her foot on his upper chest. He adjusts his position so that his knees are on either side of her hips and he is close enough to enter her.

Now the woman places her bent leg behind him while lifting the straight leg and repositioning it on his chest. As she alternates the position of her legs, which being quite close together make her vagina tight around his penis, she massages his erection. If she uses her vaginal muscles at the same time, both lovers can experience a variety of intensely pleasurable sensations.

If the woman wants to give temporary control to the man, she can stay still for a while and let the man thrust instead.

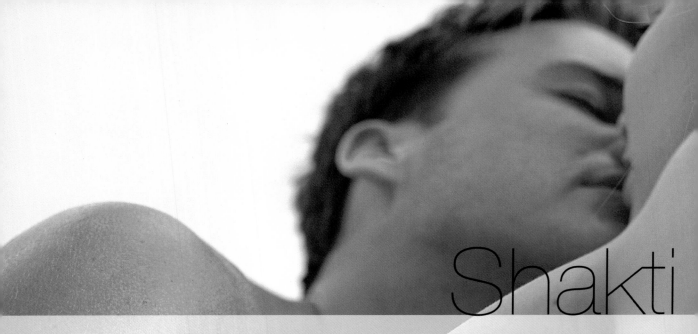

Shakti

Shakti is the deity representing the female. Her energy resides in the base *chakra* (one of the seven energy centres) sited at the perineum, between the vagina and the anus. Her partner, Shiva, who represents maleness resides in the crown *chakra* on the top of the head. This tantric position has been simplified to make it achievable by those who are not as flexible as yoga experts. But, as always, just have fun with it and adapt it to your own abilities.

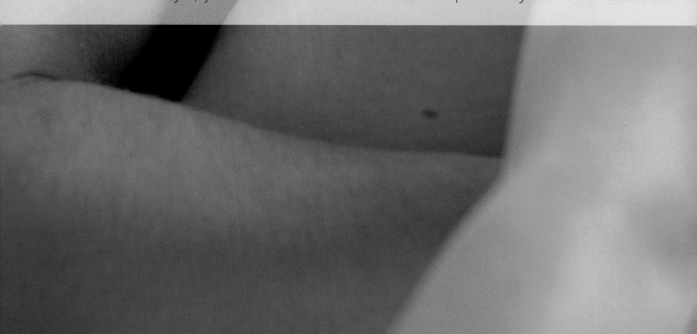

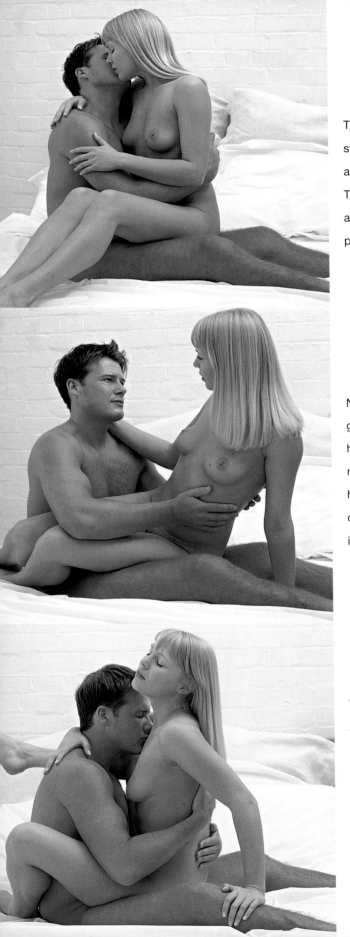

The man sits with his back straight and his legs stretched out in front of him. He can sit either on a floor cushion or, if he prefers, on a bed or sofa. The woman sits sideways on his lap, with her right arm draped around his shoulder. In this position he penetrates her.

Now the woman, keeping her legs together and gripping his penis with her vaginal muscles, bends her knees so that her feet are pointing behind the man and her knees are pointing forward, away from his body. While in this pose the couple can kiss and caress each other while she continues using her internal muscles to help him stay erect.

To take it a step further, the woman leans back and supports herself with one hand on his leg while he holds her firmly round her waist and swings her right leg over his head to rest it on his left shoulder. As you can imagine, attempting such a movement may provoke fits of laughter, but having a go and having a laugh are better for your sex life than never trying.

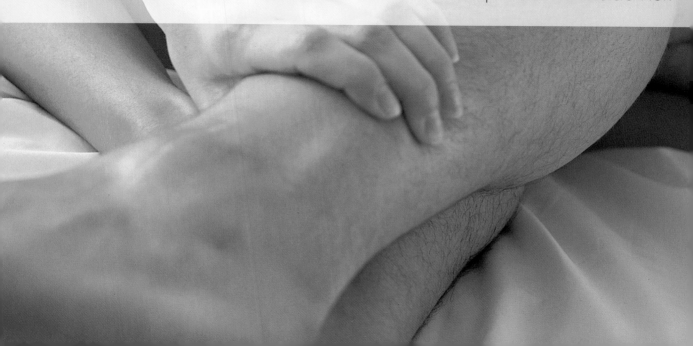

Drawing the bow

Men and women have different fantasies about early morning sex: women would like their partners to penetrate them while they are just waking up; while men would like to be awoken with oral sex. Side positions are excellent for initiating early morning sex when you might want to start slowly as you both wake up and work up to something more energetic. This position is ideal for a man to fulfil the wish of a woman who wants to wake up with him inside her.

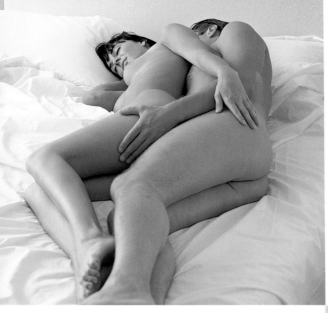

The woman lies on her side facing away from the man, while he lies close behind her facing her back.

Gently he lifts her uppermost leg and squeezes both his legs between hers. He now guides his penis into her and, holding her shoulders, pulls her slowly but firmly back towards him.

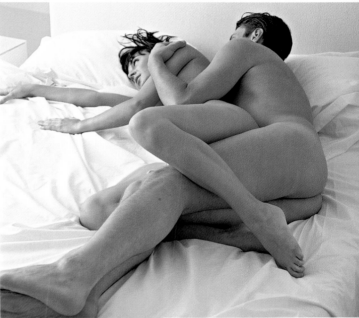

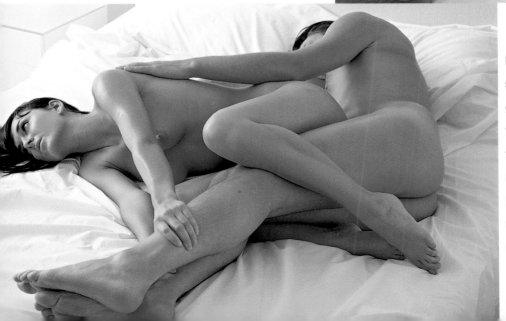

Now she is rousing, she reaches down and grabs his feet, pulling them up towards her – thus creating a bow-and-arrow shape. In this posture both lovers move together, using their hips to generate movement.

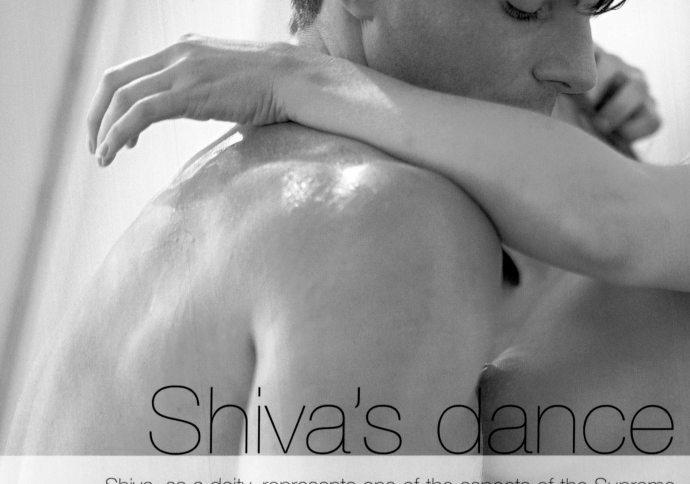

Shiva's dance

Shiva, as a deity, represents one of the aspects of the Supreme

Being. He is often depicted in the form of a phallus but can also be

seen as a many-armed dancer, which gives this standing position its

name. This 'dancing' posture can be adopted very quickly and so is

ideal for fast, energetic sex, but the stillness during penetration also

allows for moments of reflection and quiet tenderness.

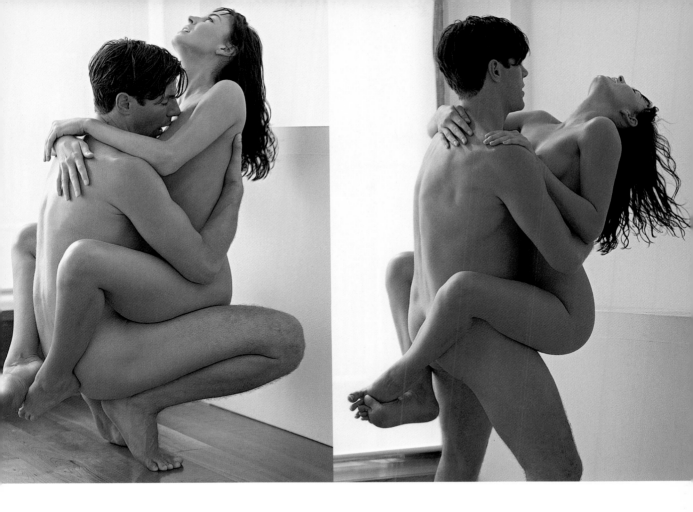

For speed and ease of adopting this posture, the woman sits on the edge of a bed or chair with her legs apart while the man squats between them. She then wraps her legs around his back. In this squatting position, he penetrates her and stands up, lifting her with him. For her part, she clasps her hands around the back of his neck and grips his waist with her thighs. Now, she can thrust against him vigorously while he supports her buttocks with his hands and guides her movements.

When one or both lovers need a break, he lowers her to a sitting position while staying inside her. Now they may want to follow the tantric practice of stillness, where they both focus on the build-up of genital sensations and sexual tension until the urge to thrust again cannot be resisted. He then lifts her again so he can carry on thrusting and finally orgasm.

Remaining still during penetration encourages lovers to become aware of their own and their partner's individual patterns of desire.

Wild abandon

This energetic position requires a good degree of suppleness and strength. Fortunately, as its name suggests, it is one in which the vigour of the movements may take lovers beyond what they thought were their physical limits, especially if they have warmed up beforehand. In this respect, sex is not dissimilar to dance or sport: when the body is warm it is more flexible and less susceptible to injury.

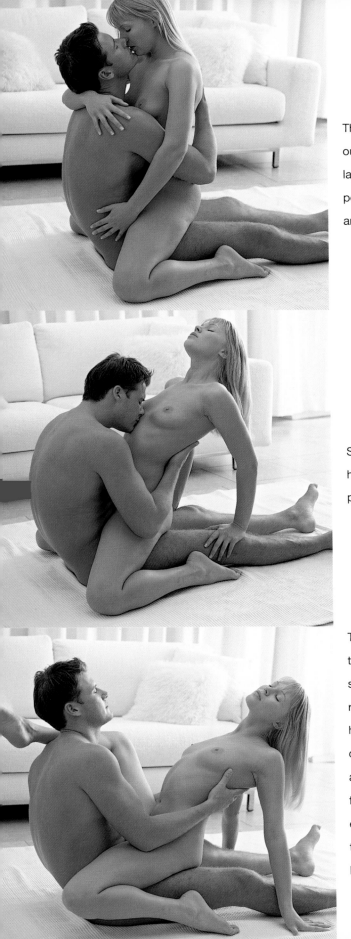

The man sits upright on the floor with his legs stretched out in front of him, while the woman kneels astride his lap, facing him, her knees gripping his hips. At this point he penetrates her and the lovers then wrap their arms around each other's backs.

She now leans back and he offers support by holding her round the waist until she can support herself by placing her palms on his legs or the floor.

The woman lifts her right leg up and swings it over the man's left shoulder. The man then leans back and supports himself on his hands. He uses this support to raise his buttocks off the floor and thrusts deeply into his partner, making his movements as strong as he can. The thrusting movements lift her body with his, although she always keeps her left foot on the ground for support. When a moment of relaxation from this energetic movement is needed, the lovers should return to the initial step of this posture, hold each other tightly, bodies close, and rock together from side to side.

Tranquil

A conscious decision to experience sex in a meditative way will allow you to align yourself more closely with your own senses, emotions and body rhythms and, importantly, with those of your partner. The use of slow movements, of listening to your breath and bringing it into harmony with your lover's, and of paying attention to your senses of touch and smell, will permit you to experience sexual arousal as a total body experience rather than one confined largely to your genitals.

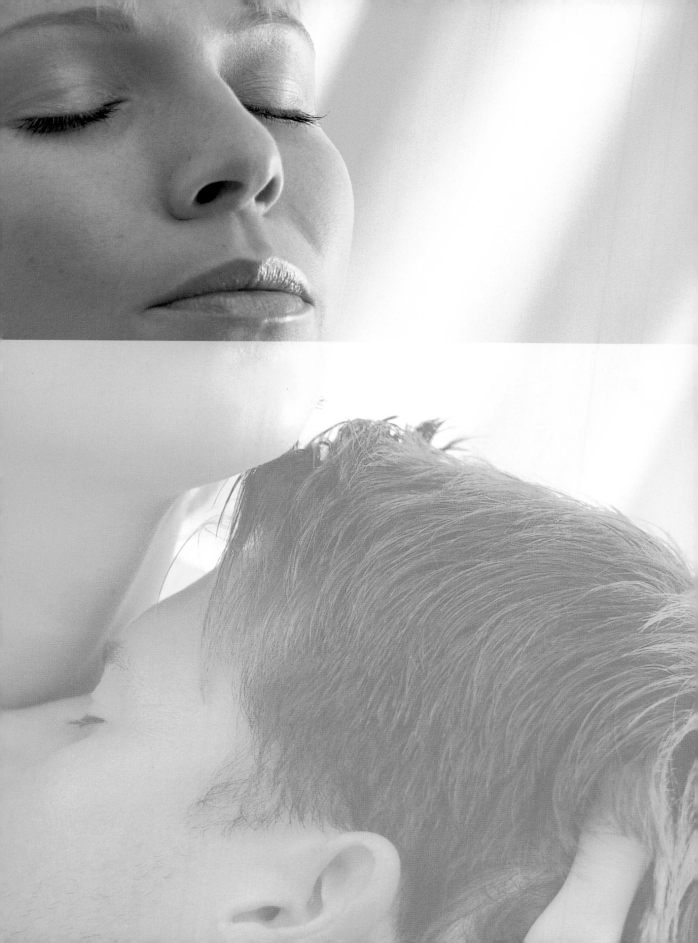

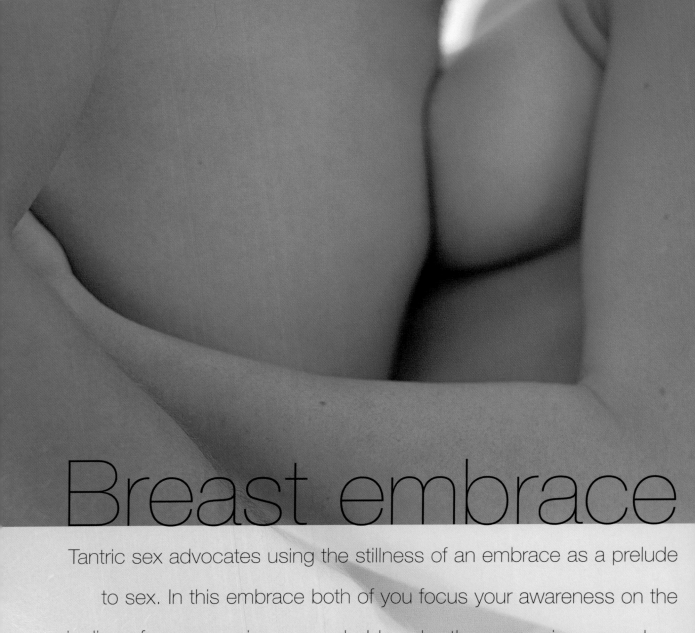

Breast embrace

Tantric sex advocates using the stillness of an embrace as a prelude to sex. In this embrace both of you focus your awareness on the mingling of your energies as you hold each other, preparing yourselves for the union of that energy in the cosmic dance of Shiva and Shakti.

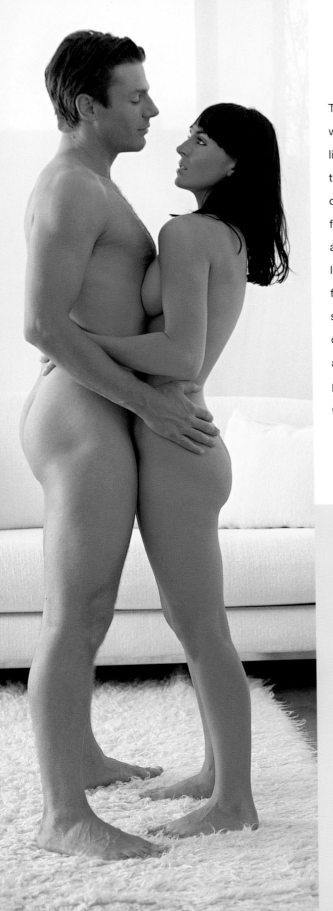

The lovers stand facing each other with open arms and warmly embrace one another. They press their bodies lightly together, making sure that they are touching at the breast, belly, pelvis and thighs. They gaze into each other's eyes, allowing their eyes to relax rather than focus, and bring their mouths close together without actually touching. Now in the embrace, they feel and listen to the rhythm of their partner's breath, which they feel spreading warmth through their bodies. Each person senses the energy of arousal this brings to many parts of their body, including the genitals. They then allow the arousal to increase slowly until both instinctively feel the point where they want to experience sexual union, then gently separate and begin.

In the tantric tradition, Shakti is the deity representing the female principle; her partner, Shiva, represents the male principle.

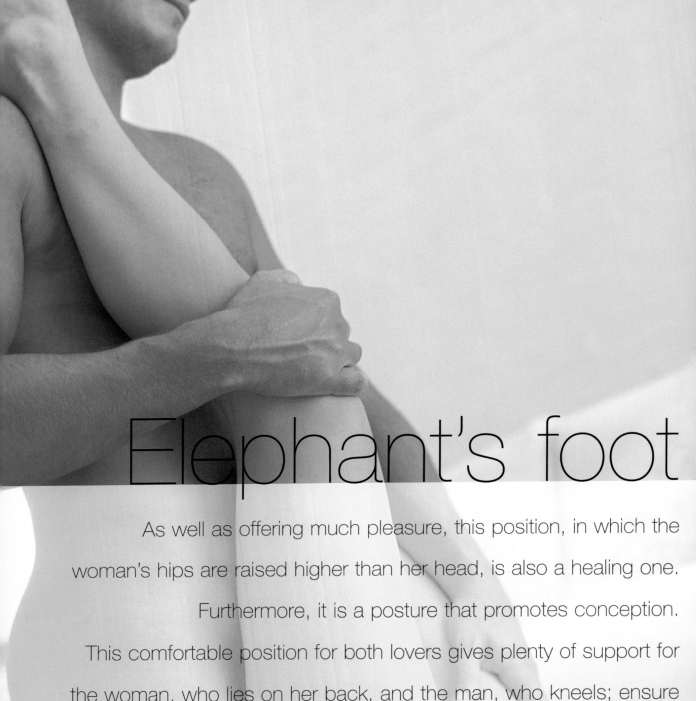

Elephant's foot

As well as offering much pleasure, this position, in which the
woman's hips are raised higher than her head, is also a healing one.
Furthermore, it is a posture that promotes conception.
This comfortable position for both lovers gives plenty of support for
the woman, who lies on her back, and the man, who kneels; ensure
there are enough cushions or pillows nearby to enhance comfort.

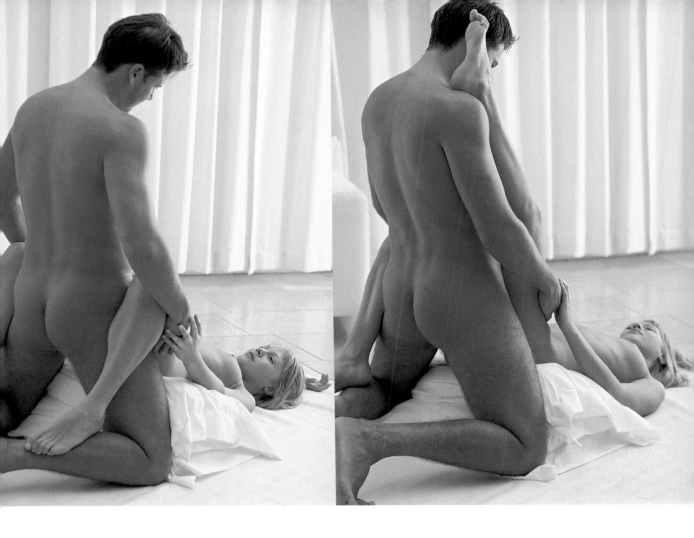

To set the scene, the woman lies on her back with her head on a pillow if wished. The man squeezes some pillows under her hips, one at a time, until they are raised higher than her head and high enough to be nearly level with his genitals when he is kneeling.

The man, kneeling between her thighs, places one of her legs over his shoulder. Now he enters her and alternates deep and shallow thrusting, while also being able to play with her clitoris at the same time. As her lower back is well supported, she should be comfortable staying in this posture for some time, allowing him to pleasure her without feeling she has to do anything whatsoever.

The pleasurable sensations come from the alternating deep and shallow thrusting.

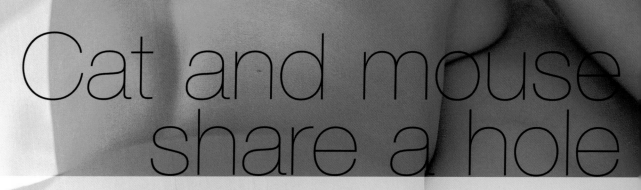

Cat and mouse
share a hole

There are times when one or both lovers want a break

during energetic sex. This woman-on-top posture still allows

deep penetration while, at the same time, providing the woman

with a lot of clitoral stimulation. It is also a fantastic position to try

if one or both partners are having difficulty reaching orgasm;

alternating between vigorous thrusting and this posture

allows both partners to focus on genital sensations.

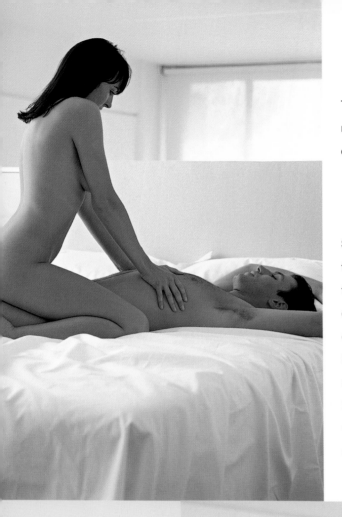

The man lies on his back with his legs straight but relaxed. The woman sits astride him and guides herself down on to his erect penis.

She then lowers her body on to his: her legs lie along the top of his, her upper body is supported on her forearms but lies along his torso, and her hands rest on or under his shoulders. He may wish to rest his hands on her buttocks, gently guiding her movements. While holding his shoulders, she can move gently up and down or, together, they may roll from side to side. By doing this, she can control her clitoral stimulation while using her vaginal muscles to increase stimulation of her partner's penis.

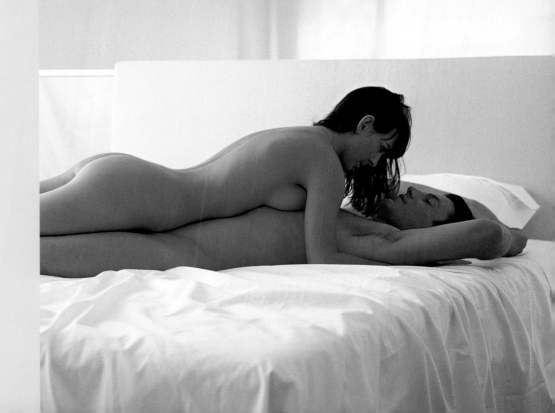

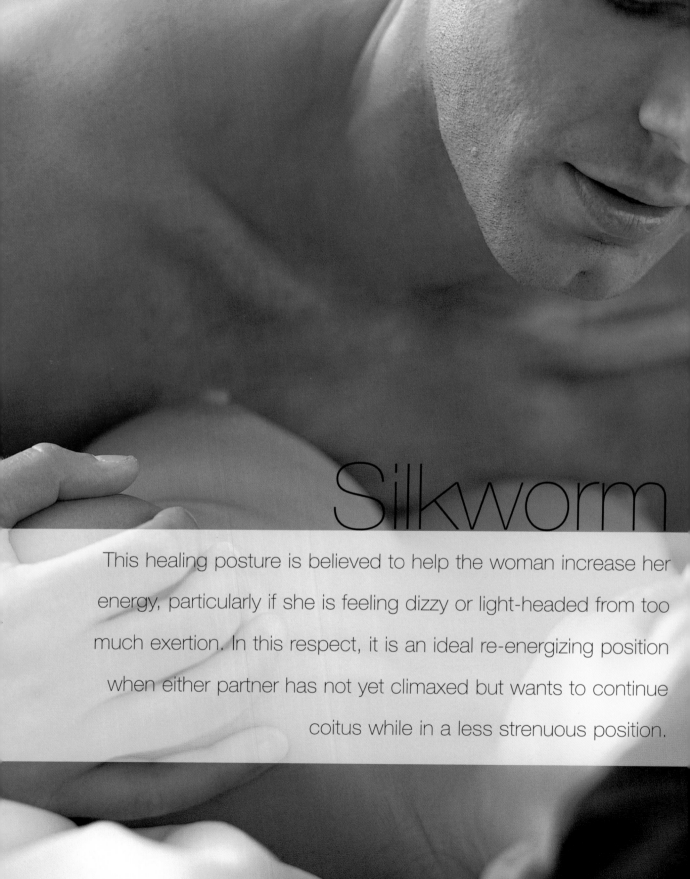

Silkworm

This healing posture is believed to help the woman increase her energy, particularly if she is feeling dizzy or light-headed from too much exertion. In this respect, it is an ideal re-energizing position when either partner has not yet climaxed but wants to continue coitus while in a less strenuous position.

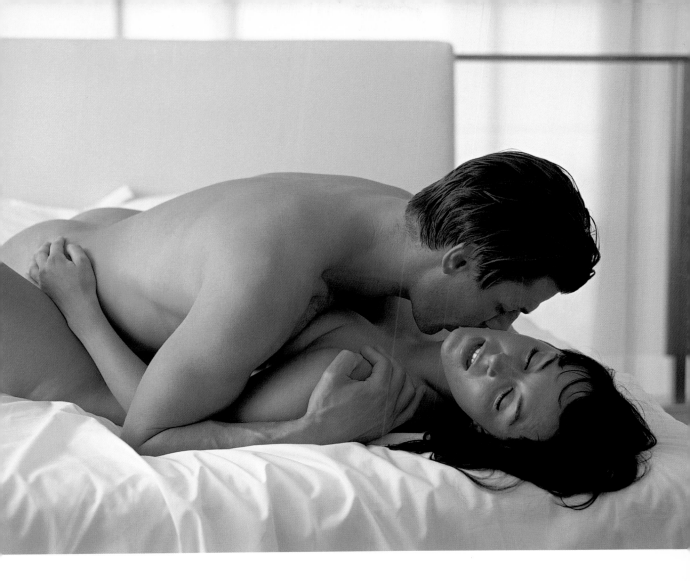

To start with the couple adopts the famous Missionary position (see page 12) with the woman lying on her back and the man lying on top of her. He penetrates her deeply and lies along her body, cupping her shoulders in his hands. She now rhythmically rotates her pelvis, alternating between clockwise and anticlockwise directions. These gyrations, in effect, act as an internal massage, stimulating various acupressure points around the penis. The woman continues to slowly gyrate her hips until one or both partners climax.

This sexual healing position can also help lovers boost their energy levels.

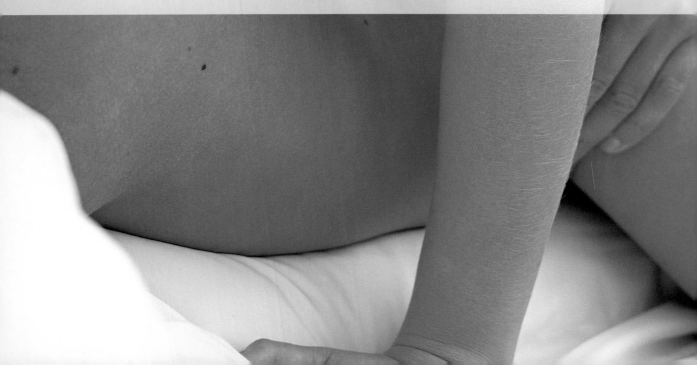

Elephant posture

This rear-entry position combines relaxation with deep penetration. With the strategic use of cushions or pillows, lovers can move from a position like The Plough (see page 78), for example, or another rear-entry position where the woman's back and hips can become strained, to this resting posture without the man having to withdraw.

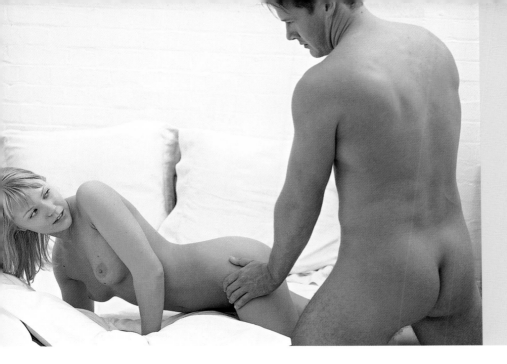

The woman lies on her belly, with her head resting on a pillow and her arms relaxed in a comfortable position. A cushion slipped under her belly or pelvis will raise her hips slightly.

The man penetrates her and lies his body along the length of her back, at the same time supporting himself with one hand on the bed and the other on her hip, so that she is not taking too much of his weight. If moving into this position from another, it should be easy to maintain penetration as long as both partners' movements are controlled. The emphasis is on slow thrusting, just fast enough to keep both lovers aroused.

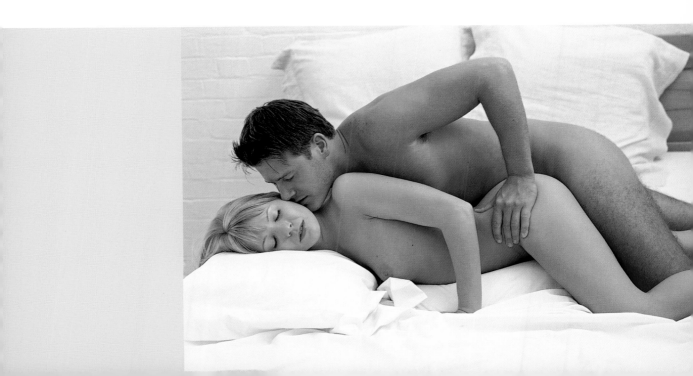

Yawning posture

The name of this posture refers to yawning in the sense of being wide open. In this pose, the woman can maintain absolute stillness while the man controls the movements. It is ideal for any woman who finds it difficult to move her hips while on her back or who has a lower-back problem.

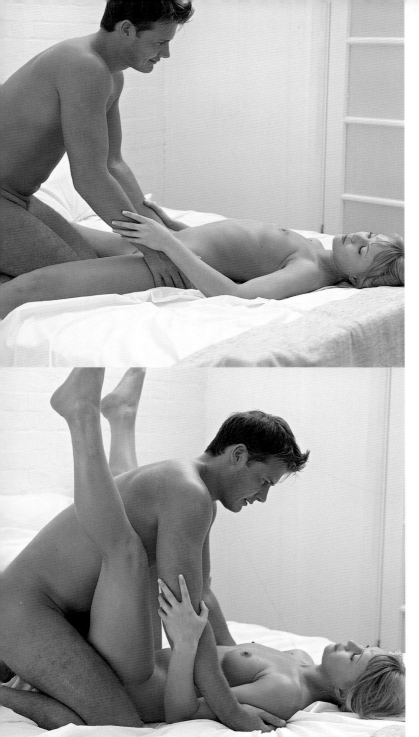

The woman lies on her back with her head supported by a pillow. She spreads her legs and keeps them outstretched and straight. The man kneels close to her, placing his knees on either side of her hips. From here, she can rest her legs on top of his thighs, while keeping them straight and pointing her toes so as to make a V-shape.

While supporting himself on his hands, placed either side of his partner, he penetrates her. He varies his thrusting movements, thus intensifying both his and his partner's sensations. Meanwhile, if she finds it a strain to keep her legs straight, she can vary her position by bending her legs at the knees, by crossing them around his back or in any other way she finds pleasurable.

Although the man is in control of movement, the woman still plays an active role by using her internal muscles.

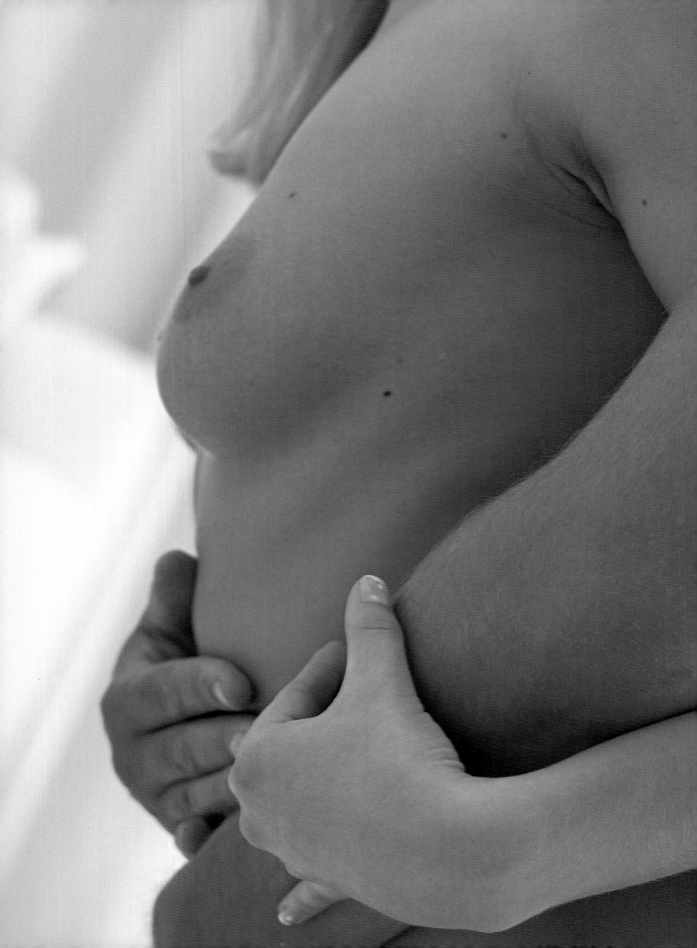

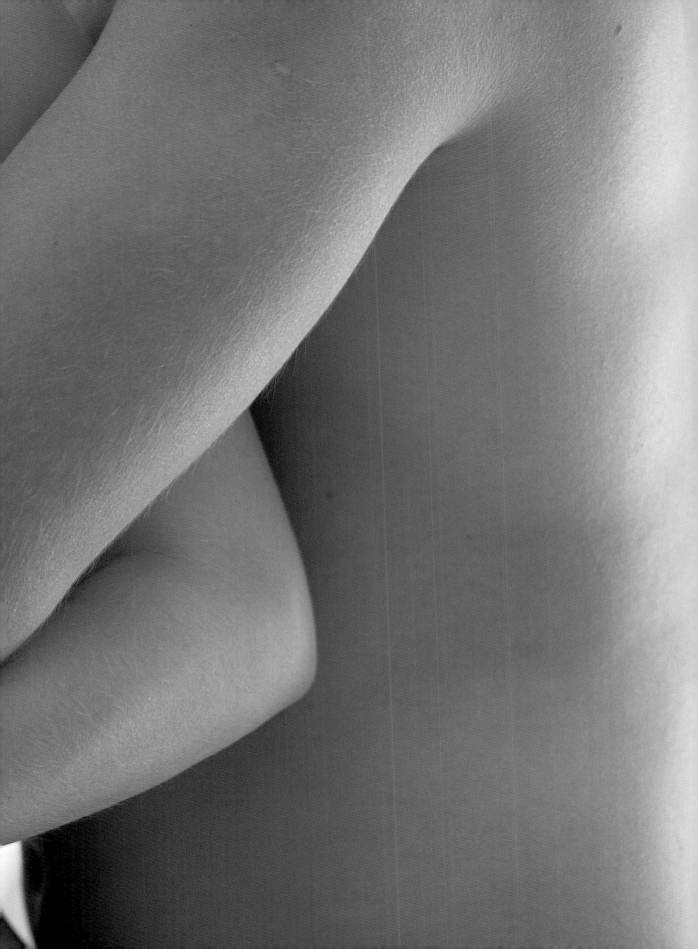

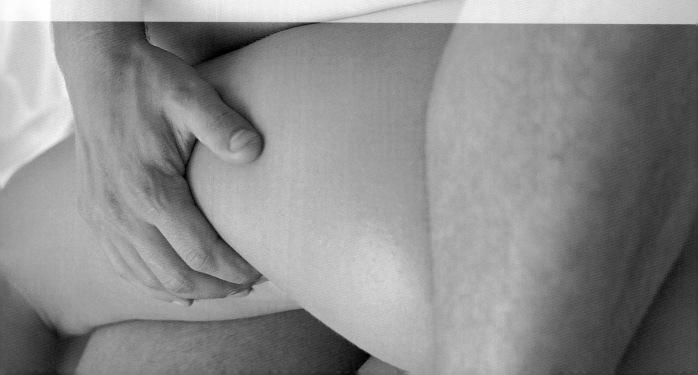

The fusion of love

In the dance of Shiva and Shakti, the ultimate aim is the fusion of the two opposing, but equal, qualities to create a whole entity. This posture can give both partners a sense of balance, in that neither one is in a superior position. There is a closeness of genital contact without movement that creates its own form of pleasure.

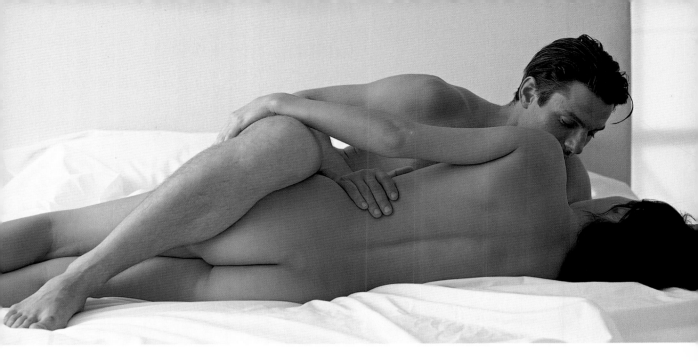

The lovers lie on their sides facing each other, their genitals touching. The man keeps his lower leg straight and lifts his other leg, wrapping it gently around the woman's hip.

From this intimate posture, he enters her and firmly pulls her upper leg towards his buttocks. In doing this he may arch his upper body away from hers so that he can penetrate her more fully and deeply. He may thrust into her or, alternatively, they can move their hips together in circular or back-and-forth motions that also provide added clitoral stimulation.

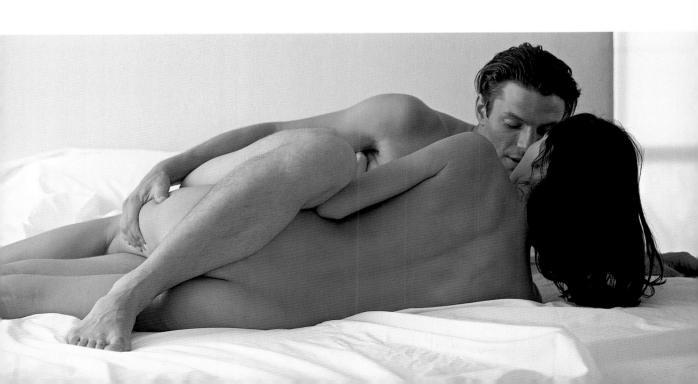

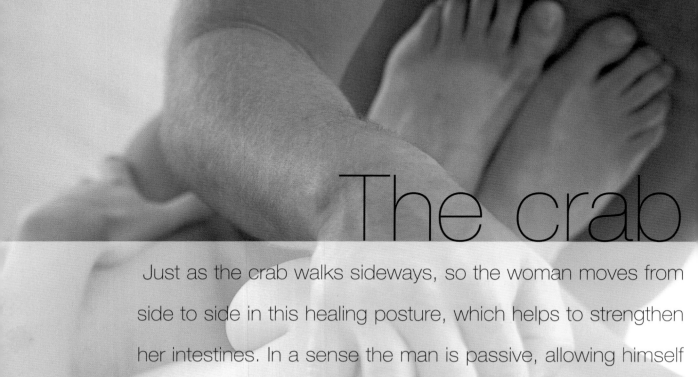

The crab

Just as the crab walks sideways, so the woman moves from side to side in this healing posture, which helps to strengthen her intestines. In a sense the man is passive, allowing himself to be 'used' by the woman as an instrument of her pleasure. His pleasure comes from hers. There is an understanding that sex is a process of give and take until both are completely satisfied.

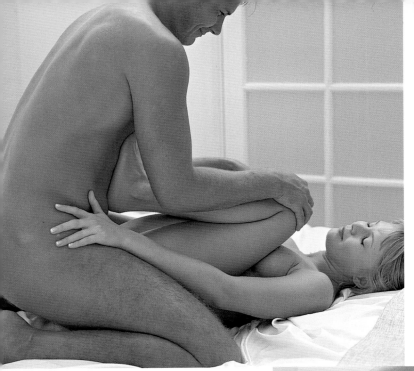

The woman lies on her back, without raising her head, and bends her knees up to her chest. The man kneels in front of her and enters her. Holding her knees, he rubs them against her breasts. With her knees raised, her vagina is tightened around his penis and he need only use gentle, shallow thrusting movements.

Now, the man releases her knees. The woman puts the soles of her feet together and rests them against his body. Her legs fall open a little in this posture and then she rocks from side to side. Alternating between these postures prolongs the man's erection so that both lovers experience a variety of sensations.

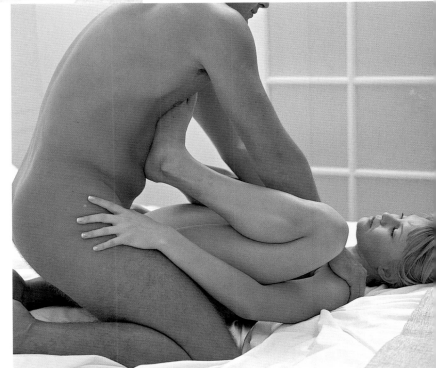

In any healthy sexual partnership there is a strong element of one partner deriving satisfaction solely from the other's enjoyment.

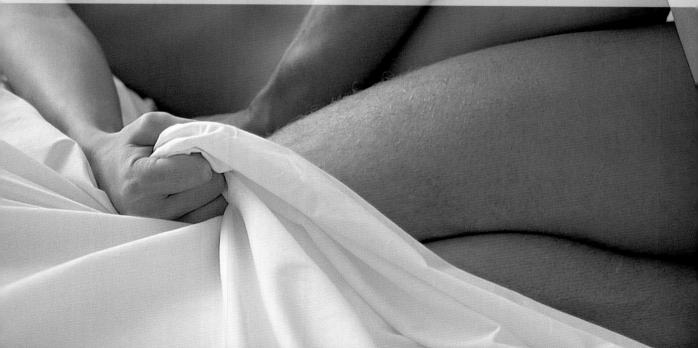

The spear

Although the name of this position undoubtedly creates a phallic image in the mind, it is a gentle, reflective posture in which the couple can focus on subtle sensations. It is also a position that the woman can adapt, depending on how athletic or supple she is, by either balancing her straightened leg on the man's head or placing her bent leg on his shoulder.

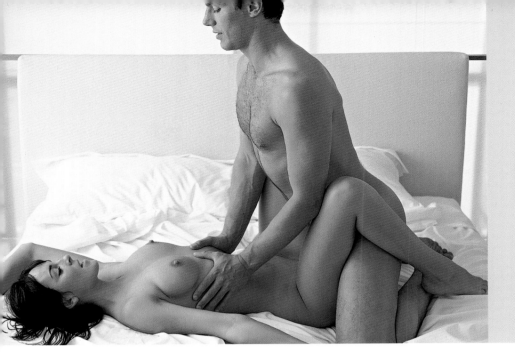

As the woman lies on her back on the bed the man kneels down between her legs, facing her. She hooks her legs over his thighs, her knees bent.

While keeping one leg bent, she raises her other leg (with his help) and rests it lightly on top of his shoulder or, according to the ancient text, his head; he may need to lean forward and lower his position so that this is possible. He can then enter her and thrust into her slowly.

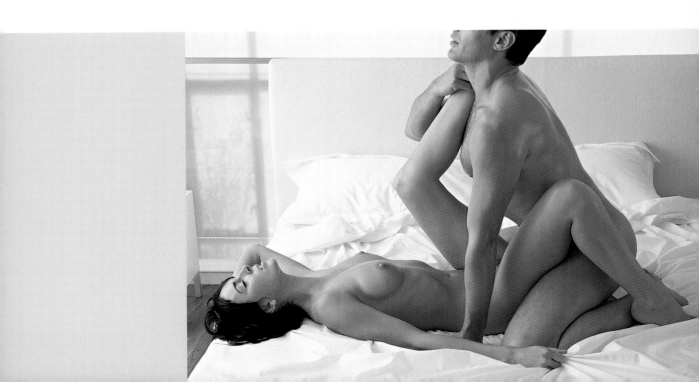

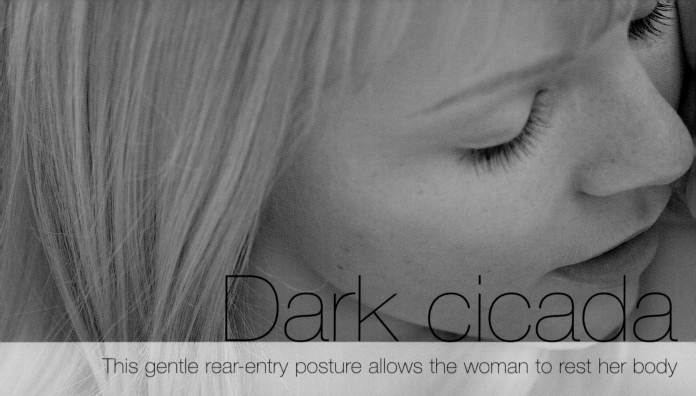

Dark cicada

This gentle rear-entry posture allows the woman to rest her body completely while still permitting the man to penetrate her deeply, if desired. It is a particularly good position to adopt if the woman is having problems with lower-back pain, as she does not bear any weight on her spine nor make any movements that might jar it. It is also a good position for G-spot stimulation.

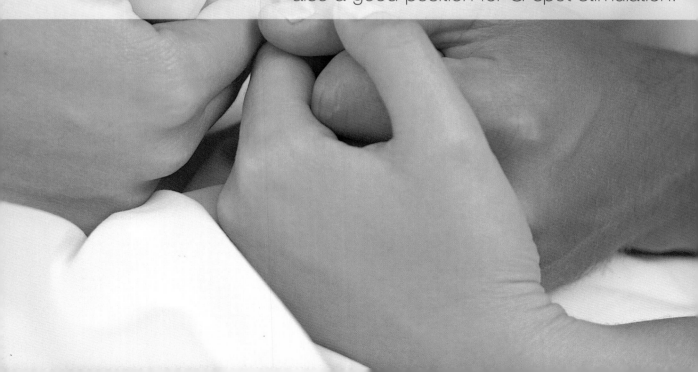

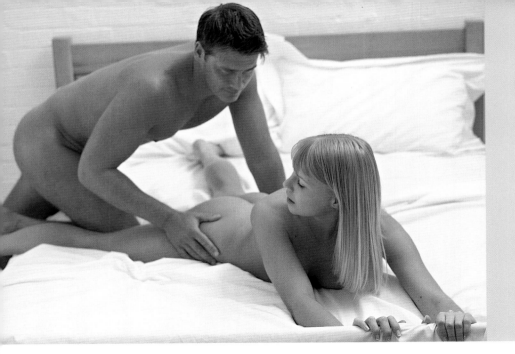

The woman lies flat on the bed on her belly, with her head supported by a pillow if she wishes. She then spreads her legs as far apart as is comfortable for her.

The man penetrates her from behind and supports his weight on his forearms, ensuring that, although his body is close to hers, she is not bearing his weight. By lowering or raising his body he can vary the strength and depth of his thrusting, alternating thrusting with moments of stillness or gentle, shallow movements.

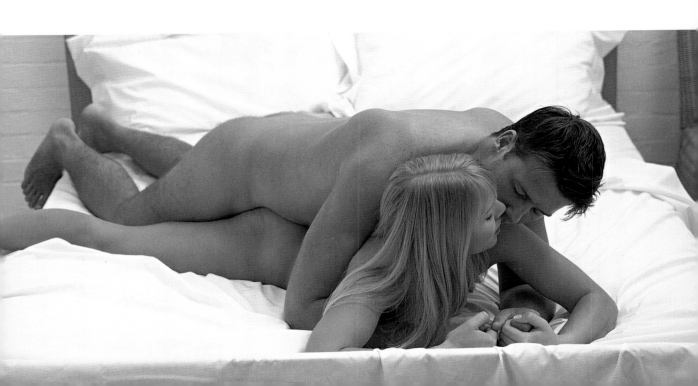

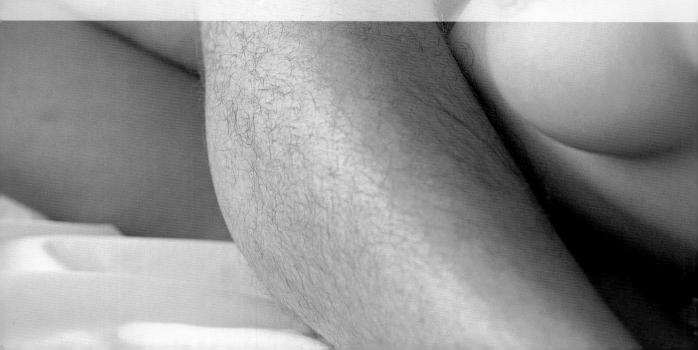

The lotus opens her petals

Although the lotus flower opens its petals in the morning, this position is not confined to pre-breakfast sex; it is perfect for resting, perhaps even for falling asleep in. In this posture the couple are joined by their genitals, their bodies falling away from each other rather than entwined as is more usual with the majority of post-coital positions.

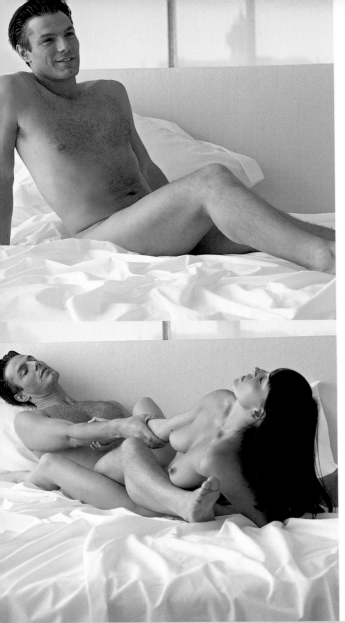

The man sits on the bed with his left leg outstretched and his right leg raised and bent at the knee, his right foot flat on the bed. He reaches behind his back and uses his hands to support himself.

The woman sits facing him and slips her left leg gently under his raised right leg. She rests her right leg over his outstretched left leg and then leans back on her hands or forearms for support. In this position he penetrates her. Now, the lovers clasp each by the right arm while leaning on the other elbow. Gradually they lean away from each other until both of them are lying flat on the bed.

The lovers release their grip and let their arms fall into a relaxed position. The woman may need to use her vaginal muscles to prevent the man from slipping out. Pleasurable sensations can be had via subtle hip movements, but this position is not suitable for any thrusting action; the emphasis is on relaxation while keeping intimate contact.

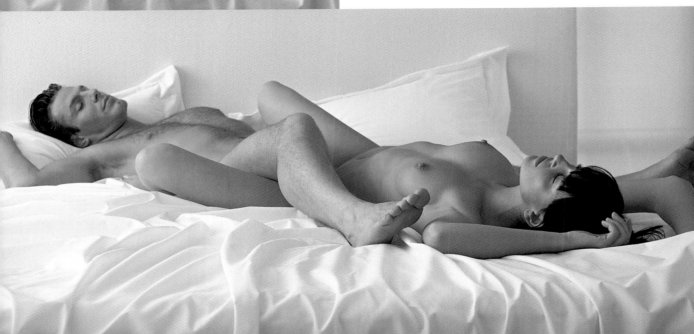

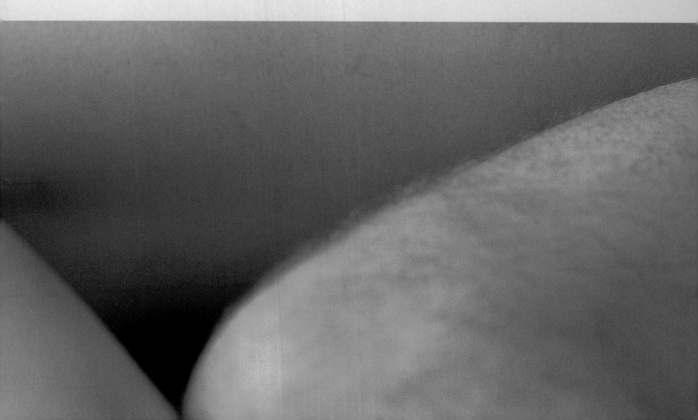

Spoons

This position is one that people fall into universally when they want to experience the feeling of closeness. Furthermore, it provides the woman with a sense of being protected, while the man enjoys the feeling of being the protector. And, if they wake in this position, the woman can enjoy feeling the man's erection against her buttocks, arousing her desire for some early morning sex.

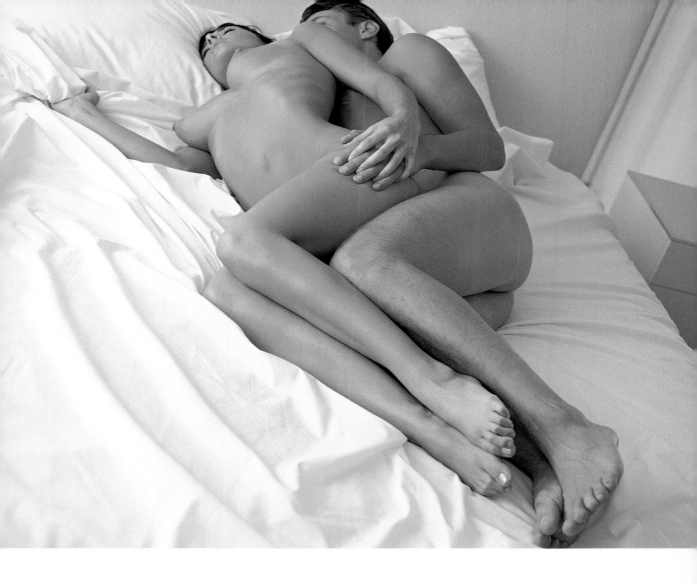

This position is so instinctive it barely requires description. The woman lies in a semi-foetal position with the man behind her, his body curved around hers, his arm around her upper body or resting on her hips. This posture can be used as a way to create arousal: one partner focuses on the other's breathing and attunes his/her own to theirs. At the same time, each lover pays attention to the body sensations at the points where their bodies are touching; both partners should allow themselves to feel these sensations without thinking ahead to what might happen next, and instead luxuriate in them as if they were a warm bath.

Undoubtedly, this is the position in which many couples sleep, whether they have had sex or not.

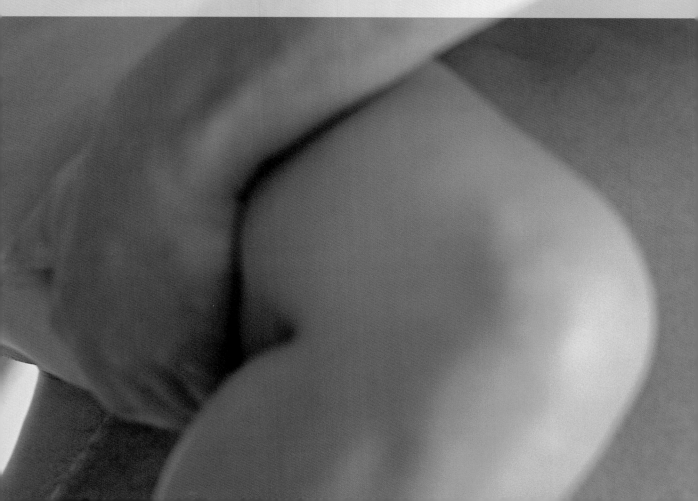

Kissing at dawn

There are times when a woman wants to show her lover how much she desires and loves him and would like to demonstrate this is in a graceful way. For new lovers or established couples, this is a simple and beautiful way to show your gratitude and devotion. The eroticism of this posture is enhanced if used after showering together or on rising before dressing. Most importantly your feet must be bare.

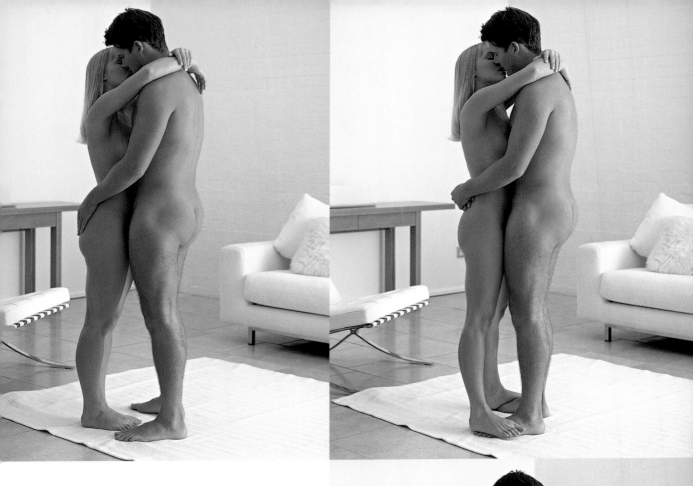

The woman approaches the man from the front and winds her arms around his neck, raising her face to look at his, her lips soft and poised to kiss him.

She then softly places the sole of her feet on top of his feet and, thus raised, kisses him deeply. This is considered a very special form of salutation.

If she wishes, she can raise one leg and wind it around the back of his upper thigh, as if she was climbing him like a tree. Take the time with this kiss so that it is arousing or, if there is no time for sex, treat it as a token of affection and a promise of pleasure to be enjoyed at a later point.

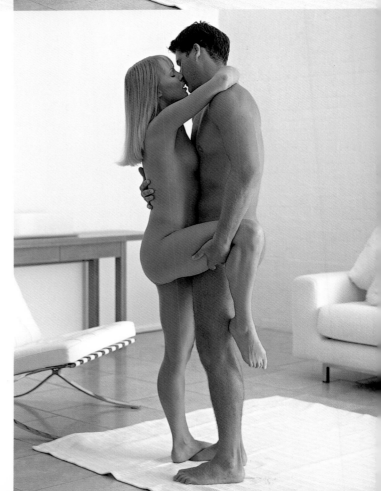

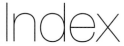

acknowledgements

Thanks to the following: Jane and Jessica at Hamlyn; Nigel, Janeanne, Reuben and the models for making it happen and having a sense of humour; the Barcelona chair for looking beautiful; the yummy cakes and crisps, which Reuben and Jessica ate, and everyone for keeping it real.

Executive Editor Jane McIntosh
Project Editor Jessica Cowie
Executive Art Editor and Designer Jo MacGregor
Art Direction Nigel Wright at XAB Design
Photography Janeanne Gilchrist at Unit Photographic
Senior Production Controller Manjit Sihra